Young Citizens in the Digital Age

A social anxiety currently pervades the political classes of the western world, arising from the perception that young people have become disaffected with liberal democratic politics. Voter turnout among 18- to 25-year-olds continues to be lower than other age groups and they are less likely to join political parties. This is not, however, proof that young people are not interested in politics per se but is evidence that they are becoming politically socialised within a new media environment. This shift poses a significant challenge to politicians who increasingly have to respond to a technologically mediated lifestyle politics that celebrates lifestyle diversity, personal disclosure and celebrity. This book explores alternative approaches for engaging and understanding young people's political activity and looks at the adoption of ICTs as a means to facilitate the active engagement of young people in democratic societies. Questions asked include:

- How important is the Internet for young people's civic and political engagement?
- What evidence exists for new media to offer the prospect of stimulating new forms of mobilization by young citizens themselves?
- How might the ICTs be used in citizenship education?
- Are new media styles of political communication required to reconnect with the interests of contemporary youth culture?

Young Citizens in the Digital Age presents new research and the first comprehensive analysis of ICTs, citizenship and young people from an international group of leading scholars. It is an important book for students and researchers of citizenship and ICTs within the fields of sociology, politics, social policy, media studies and communication studies among others.

Brian D. Loader is Co-Director of the Social Informatics Research Unit at the University of York, UK. He has written extensively on new media and socio-political and cultural change.

Young Citizens in the Digital Age

Political engagement, young people and new media

Edited by
Brian D. Loader

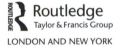
Routledge
Taylor & Francis Group

LONDON AND NEW YORK

First published 2007
by Routledge
2 Park Square, Milton Park, Abingdon, Oxon, OX14 4RN

Simultaneously published in the USA and Canada
by Routledge
270 Madison Ave, New York, NY10016

*Routledge is an imprint of the Taylor & Francis Group,
an informa business*

Typeset in Times New Roman by
Florence Production Ltd, Stoodleigh, Devon
Printed and bound in Great Britain by
TJ International Ltd, Padstow, Cornwall

British Library Cataloguing in Publication Data
A catalogue record for this book is available
from the British Library

Library of Congress Cataloging in Publication Data
Young citizens in the digital age: political engagement, young
people, and new media/edited by Brian D. Loader.
       p. cm.
     Includes bibliographical references and index.
  1. Young adults – Political activity.   2. Youth – Political
  activity.   3. Internet – Political aspects.   4. Political participation.
  5. Political socialization.   I. Loader, Brian, 1958–
  HQ799.9.P6Y67 2007
  320.0835 – dc22   2006100338

ISBN10: 0–415–40913–6 (hbk)
ISBN10: 0–415–40912–8 (pbk)
ISBN10: 0–203–94672–3 (ebk)

ISBN13: 978–0–415–40913–1 (hbk)
ISBN13: 978–0–415–40912–4 (pbk)
ISBN13: 978–0–203–94672–5 (ebk)

In memory and gratitude
Professor Jon Clark
1949–2005
Distinguished scholar and teacher

Contents

Notes on contributors

Roger Austin is Head of the School of Education at the University of Ulster and has published extensively on the role of ICT in history, teacher training and intercultural education. He is co-director of the Dissolving Boundaries Programme, which is using video-conferencing and computer conferencing to link 180 schools in Northern Ireland and the Republic of Ireland.

W. Lance Bennett is Professor of Political Science and Ruddick C. Lawrence Professor of Communication (http://faculty.washington.edu) and Director of the Centre for Communication and Civic Engagement, University of Washington (http://www.engagedcitizen.org).

Davide Calenda is Professor in Techniques of Communication and Networking at the Political Science Faculty and Research Assistant for a multidisciplinary research programme at the University of Florence, which involves Computer Science, Political Science, Law and Economy.

Stephen Coleman is Professor of Political Communication at the University of Leeds. He has written extensively on aspects of e-participation, including a recent study, *Remixing Citizenship: Democracy and Young People's Use of the Internet,* published in 2005 by the Carnegie Young People's Initiative.

Nick Couldry is Professor of Media and Communications at Goldsmiths College and was previously Reader in Media, Communications and Culture at the London School of Economics. He is the author or editor of six books, most recently *Listening Beyond the Echoes: Media, Ethics and Agency in an Uncertain World* (Paradigm Books, 2006).

Peter Dahlgren is Professor of Media and Communication at Lund University, Sweden. His recent work focuses on democracy, culture, identity and the media, with an emphasis on the media's role in contributing to democratic participation.

Ross Ferguson is New Media Manager and Director of e-Democracy at the Hansard Society. Ross is responsible for working with citizens, parliamentarians and the media to encourage greater participation in the democratic process through new technologies.

Roman Gerodimos is Associate Lecturer and doctoral candidate at the Centre for Public Communication Research, Bournemouth Media School.

Sonia Livingstone is Professor of Social Psychology in the Department of Media and Communications at the London School of Economics and Political Science. Her current work concerns domestic, familial and educational contexts of new media access, use and regulation. Recent books include *Audiences and Publics* (Intellect, 2005) and *The Handbook of New Media* (Sage, 2006).

Brian D. Loader is Co-Director of the Social Informatics Research Unit which is based in the Department of Sociology at the University York. He is editor of the international journal *Information, Communication and Society* (Taylor & Francis, Routledge) and has published widely and given presentations on the area of social and political informatics.

Tim Markham is Lecturer in Media (Journalism) in the Faculty of Continuing Education, Birkbeck College, University of London. Previously he was Research Officer in the Department of Media and Communications, London School of Economics. His research has examined war correspondence in relation to the sociology of journalism and the rise of the journalist as moral authority.

Gustavo S. Mesch is a Senior Lecturer in the Department of Sociology and Anthropology and a Senior Research Associate at the Minerva Center of Youth Studies at the University of Haifa, Israel. He studies patterns of Internet use and the role of the Internet in adolescents' social networks online and offline.

Lorenzo Mosca is Research Assistant at the European University Institute of Florence, in the DEMOS project (Democracy in Europe and the Mobilization of Society): http://demos.iue.it/

Tobias Olsson is researcher at Lund University, where he works on the EU project, Young People, the Internet and Civic Participation. He has published a number of journal articles, book chapters and reports on this theme, and has made several presentations at international conferences. He is also a lecturer in Media and Communication Studies at Växjö University.

Neil Selwyn is a Senior Lecturer at the London Knowledge Lab, University of London, where his research focuses on technology, society and education. The two overriding themes throughout his work are the place of technology in everyday life and the sociology of educational technology. Recent books include *Adult Learning in the Digital Age*

(Routledge, 2005), *Telling Tales on Technology* (Ashgate, 2002) and *The Information Age* (UWP, 2002).

Ariadne Vromen is a Lecturer in Government and International Relations at the University of Sydney. Her research and teaching interests are in the broad field of political sociology.

Janelle Ward is currently a PhD candidate at the Amsterdam School of Communication Research (ASCoR), University of Amsterdam. Her research interests include young people, citizenship and political youth websites.

Michael Xenos is an Assistant Professor of Communication Arts at the University of Wisconsin-Madison. His research interests are in political communication, with emphases on communication technology and democratic deliberation.

Preface

The level of political participation and civic engagement in a society can be seen as a measure of the health of the democratic body politic. Its future and continuing well-being falls on the shoulders of its youngest citizens and it is therefore of particular interest to the citizen and politician alike to know how committed young people are to democratic politics. Survey and polling results indicate that young people are disaffected with traditional democratic institutions and practices in many countries around the world. But the picture of apathy becomes more complicated when the experiences of young people are considered within the context of growing up in a rapidly changing socio-economic world characterised by globalisation, individualisation, deinstitutionalisation, increased mobility, consumerism, and saturated by new media such as the Internet. Many of the familiar social institutions and communication channels that have traditionally facilitated political socialisation can no longer be regarded as stable factors shaping young people's identities as citizens. Such changing social circumstances may alternatively act to disguise the level of political interest of young people who may be more easily committed to single-issue campaigns and the politics of lifestyle, environment, global justice, anti-poverty, and what some have described as the 'identity project' (Giddens, 1991), which find less favour among parliamentary debates and political party manifestoes.

In a world increasingly influenced by the Internet, World Wide Web, iPods and texting, it is perhaps unsurprising that these new media are seen as playing an important role in the debate about young people and civic engagement. For some, the new media are a part of the problem and both provide escapist distractions as well as undermining serious deliberation. Yet for others, information and communications technologies (ICTs) provide the solution for reconnecting young people with politics. This collection, which is the outcome of a small symposium of international scholars hosted by the Social Informatics Research Unit based at the Department of Sociology, University of York, in September 2005, is intended to make a contribution to this debate. It attempts to address a number of questions. How important is the Internet for young people's civic and political engagement? What evidence exists for new media to offer the prospect of stimulating new forms of mobilisation by young citizens themselves? How might ICTs be used in citizenship education? Are new media styles of political communication required to reconnect with the interests of contemporary youth culture?

My thanks go to all the participants at the symposium who helped to make it such an enjoyable and stimulating occasion. I would also like to thank my colleague Roger Burrows for all his help and enthusiasm both up to and during the event itself. As always my most valued acknowledgement goes to my wife Kim and our sons William and Christopher for their unerring support and forbearance.

Brian D. Loader
Ingleby Arncliffe, North Yorkshire
2006

Acknowledgements

The chapter by Sonia Livingstone, Nick Couldry and Tim Markham reports on research funded by two Economic and Social Research Council grants – *UK Children Go Online* (RES-335–25–0008), part of the 'e-Society' Programme (with co-funding from AOL, BSC, Childnet-International, Citizens Online, ITC and Ofcom; see www.children-go-online.net) and *Media Consumption and the Future of Public Connection* (RES-143–25–0011), part of the ESRC/AHRC Cultures of Consumption programme (see www.publicconnection.org). Peter Dahlgren and Tobias Olsson wish to acknowledge a generous grant from the LearnIT Research School in Sweden that made the research and their chapter possible. Davide Calenda and Lorenzo Mosca are grateful to Donatella della Porta and Brian Loader for their comments on a previous version of this paper. We thank Vittorio Mete for useful comments on the introduction and Erika Cellini, David Parlanti and Claudius Wagemann for their help on the data analysis. English was revised by Louisa Parks. The ESF survey was directed by Donatella della Porta, and coordinated by Massimiliano Andretta and Lorenzo Mosca; data inputting was managed by Maria Fabbri. The UF survey was directed by Davide Calenda and supported by Nicola Malloggi. A special thank-you goes to Dino Giuli and Marco Bontempi for their encouragement. Stephen Coleman would like to thank Janelle Ward of the University of Amsterdam for her diligent and enthusiastic contribution to this research during the 2005 election campaign; to Stephan Shakespeare and his colleagues at YouGov for running the surveys; to Peter Bazalgette, Chief Executive of Endemol, for being a supportive critic; and to participants in the York symposium for inspiring me to continue thinking through these ideas.

1 Introduction

Young citizens in the digital age: disaffected or displaced?

Brian D. Loader

Few parents nowadays pay any regard to what their children say to them. The old fashioned respect for the young is fast dying out.
Lady Bracknell: *The Importance of Being Earnest*, Act 1, Oscar Wilde.

There's nothing wrong with the younger generation that becoming taxpayers won't cure.

Dan Bennett, attributed remark

A social anxiety seems to pervade the political classes of the western world that arises from the perception that younger people have become disaffected with liberal democratic politics (Henn, 2002). The traditional mechanisms of political socialisation, which have introduced each new generation to the institutions, mores and practices of democratic governance, no longer seem to inspire commitment or engender dutiful participation. Reluctance to vote at elections and a rising average age of the membership of political parties are cited as examples of this alarming lack of engagement by young people in public affairs. Such trends are compounded by attitude surveys that reveal high levels of distrust in politicians and politics held by young people (Dalton, 2004). Paradoxically, such disenchantment comes at a time when young people are more exposed to political information and discourse through the media and education than their parents experienced. Yet this generational malaise is often interpreted as a continuation of the growing political apathy and withdrawal from public activity that is leading to a weakening of democratic citizenship in many countries worldwide.

Running counter to this pessimistic *disaffected citizen* perspective, however, one can also increasingly detect what I will describe as a *cultural displacement* perspective of young people's political engagement. This alternative view suggests that young people are not necessarily any less interested in politics than previous generations but rather that traditional political activity no longer appears appropriate to address the concerns associated with contemporary youth culture. Instead, the restricted democratic practices of voting and social class party allegiance, which have formed the basic means of collective mobilisation, are being displaced by mechanisms and modes of democratic expression that privilege present-day political preoccupations with the construction of self-identity (Giddens, 1991) within a global information economy (Castells, 1997). In this scenario it is not young people who have become disaffected with politics but rather that our political representatives appear distant and self-absorbed and unable to empathise with young people's experiences of a dramatically changing social and cultural world. Nowhere, perhaps, is this more apparent than in the gulf that is depicted between the traditional style of political communication of elected representatives and the more new media-oriented life experiences of many young people, characterised by sociological patterns of increasing fluidity, mobility, individualisation and consumerism.

The concerns of proponents of the *cultural displacement* perspective have turned to considerations of the means by which young people may become politically socialised within a media environment that celebrates lifestyle diversity, personal disclosure, and self-help therapy. Parliamentary and congressional forums, voting booths and the restrictions of social class-based party allegiance contrast strongly with the self-expression induced communication spaces of *MySpace*, *MSN*, *Flickr* and mobile texting as potential means to enable young people's political efficacy. Moreover, in a social world where celebrity, reality television and chat shows attract significantly larger audiences than civic and political association membership, such spaces may offer contexts for debates and awareness of lifestyle politics focused on sexuality, identity, environment, consumerism, gender and global justice. Indeed, it may even be possible to discern a fashionable portrayal of the young 'Internet generation' as the forerunners of an emerging techno-social and political culture. Born wired into the digital world, inhabiting the virtual spaces of online chat rooms, nurtured by the blogosphere and nourished by the flows of digital sounds and sights, these young people are seen to be significant actors shaping the parameters of democratic governance in late modern society.

From the alternative perspective of the *disaffected citizen* such a cultural turn is more often greeted with derision. From their position the socio-technical changes, while acknowledged, are largely overstated by the displacement view and do not require a significant break from existing political style. Instead, the new media can be assimilated as a new additional channel of political communication to young people about existing democratic institutions and practices. Websites, podcasts and online discussion forums can be designed to facilitate more 'modern' ways for politicians, political parties and educationists to connect with young citizens. Indeed, a mixture of citizenship education in schools and a range of initiatives which have ICTs embedded in them has been a common response to the perceived civic apathy of young people in many countries. Together with occasional appearances on talk shows by politicians and the disclosure of their iPod playlists to demonstrate their affinity with youth culture, little else is required from political representatives to reconnect with young people.

Emergent tensions and issues

These two approaches do not of course represent the only interpretations that can be made and such a sharp distinction as presented here, it may be argued, is much narrower in practice and could be fruitfully replaced with a view which foregrounds their convergence. Nonetheless, the conceptual cleavage remains helpful for placing a number of important issues in relief and opening up the debate about the possibilities of young people adopting the new media for democratic engagement. This book has the primary aim of critically exploring the role of new media in influencing the democratic acumen of young citizens in late modern societies. It is undertaken through an examination of a number of tensions that emerge between the disaffection and displacement perspectives of young people's civic engagement.

It may be useful to mention at this point some of the principle issues arising from this framework, which inform many of the contributions to this collection. First, the contrasting perspectives have a tendency to emphasise different aspects of democratic political engagement. The *citizen disaffection* perspective tends to focus upon formal institutions and procedures associated with classical liberal democratic theory such as representation, parties, parliaments and voting. Political education and communication within this framework are typically hierarchical and top-down, and shaped by idealised models of active citizenship (Combs and Nimmo, 1996). As such, they have been criticised for leaving little opportunity to hear the voice of young people or capable of enabling a sense of political efficacy. Following Murray Edelman (1971) it may be possible to regard such political socialisation as an essential introduction to the management of citizens which is practised 'not by granting or withholding their stable subjective demands, but rather by changing the demands and the expectations' (1971: 7).

The *cultural displacement* perspective attempts to widen the field of investigation to encompass deinstitutionalised forms of political engagement which are enacted within networks and spaces characterised by loose social ties and informal social structures. Here we might find *interaction* within non-hierarchical, flexible and personalised social relations, which offer the prospect of new repertoires for political socialisation outside traditional social institutions. Digital media may thereby provide young people with the communication channels to both facilitate such less regulated personal interaction and grant access to a broader range of transnational political influences. The following chapters explore how new media may influence the civic and political engagement of young people within both the formal domain of liberal democratic politics and also the informal realm of youth culture. Can the purposeful adoption of new media by politicians and political parties connect with the interests of young people? What evidence exists for new media to offer the prospect of stimulating new forms of mobilisation by young citizens themselves? How might the diffusion of ICTs shape the relationship between these two democratic domains?

A second aspect which should be mentioned before we embark upon more detailed analysis concerns what we mean by *new media*. While we are aware of the dramatic changes taking place in a wide range of digital ICTs such as mobile telephony and high resolution digital television, the primary focus of this work is the use of the Internet and World Wide Web (WWW) by young people. This includes analysis of how the Internet may influence civic engagement by young people by empirically exploring online communication. Is it different in its effect upon political socialisation from earlier forms of media? Too often, perhaps, new media theorists have been guilty of emphasising the 'newness' of the technology and the emergence of a second media age (Webster, 2001). In this volume, however, the authors have tried to be careful about jettisoning a link between old and new media and the lessons about political engagement and socialisation which may pertain to an examination of both. Young people may continue to be more influenced by television, for example, than by the Internet (Livingstone *et al.*, Chapter 2).

As well as empirical investigations of Internet usage a number of specifically designed online applications intended to engage young people are also considered. These case studies often provide examples of projects that attempt to facilitate a range of intermediate civic spaces which could exist at the interstices of the formal political institutions and the informal world of online youth culture. That is to say, they represent socio-political experiments where these two worlds can intersect at the nodes of Internet and social networks. Their design frequently begins from a recognition that young people are not a different species but, rather, share the insecurities and uncertainties arising from the global cultural transitions outlined earlier. As such, many of the lessons which may come out of these small endeavours may address the limitations of current citizenship pedagogy (see Selwyn, Chapter 9) as well as providing genuine opportunities for young people's political efficacy.

As social commentators increasingly regard the ubiquitous new media as playing an important part in the activity of engaging young citizens in democratic politics, it becomes increasingly necessary to consider the impact on this process of what is commonly referred to as the 'digital divide'. This term, more recently, has come to relate not only to unequal social access to ICTs but much more importantly to the differential use and adoption of new media (Mansell, 2002; Loader and Keeble, 2004). While lowering prices and government policies may be stimulating the expansion of online access in many countries, such crude indicators may act to disguise the socio-demographic variations in mastering the new media for political advantage. We need instead to think of youth culture as heterogeneous and contextualised in its adoption of the new media by a range of factors both facilitating and inhibiting democratic participation (see Vromen, Chapter 7). Internet use for many young people may continue to be dominated by the kind of one-dimensional communication (online shopping, downloading music and videos, online gambling) beloved of many politicians rather than the more empowering activities of personal content creation, blogging and interaction symptomatic of the *cultural* displacement model. It is as well to remember Manuel Castells' pertinent observation recognising that 'who are the *interacting* and who are the *interacted* in the new system . . . largely frames the system of domination and the processes of liberation in the informational society' (1997: 374).

Whatever the differences between the two perspectives they both seem to share an acceptance that the vitality of young people's democratic engagement in the future will be influenced by the outcomes of at least three aspects of socio-cultural transitions. These are changes in the relationship between the citizen and the nation state; the nature of civic participation; and the role of new media in the political socialisation and citizenship education of young citizens.

Globalisation, identity and the nation state

Citizenship is notoriously difficult to define. Traditionally, its locus has been derived from the nation state as a primary reference. It may encompass identity, gender, participation, attitudes, values, rights and obligations. Pattie and his colleagues approach citizenship as 'a set of norms, values and practices designed to solve collective action problems which involve the recognition by individuals that they have rights and obligations to each other if they wish to solve such problems' (Pattie *et al.*, 2004: 22). Thus citizenship comprises both attitudinal and behavioural characteristics. We consider the latter in the next section. For now we consider the normative aspect of citizenship as a set of values, symbols, experiences, imagination and identification which can provide the meaning for political action and behaviour. A familiar depiction of this dimension might be along the lines suggested by Pattie *et al.*, that it 'relates to the balance between the individual's sense of their rights and their obligations to the wider society' (ibid.). This is a useful opening at first sight until one considers what that 'wider society' might be in the light of some the most significant socio-economic changes currently underway. At least three important aspects of the current debates highlight the problematic nature of such a definition and point again to a distinction between *disaffected* and *displaced* citizenship models: globalisation and national identity; social fragmentation; and individualisation.

Globalisation and national identity

David Held describes globalisation simply as 'a shift or transformation in the scale of human organization that links distant communities and expands the reach of power relations across the world's regions' (2004: 1). At a time when many such commentators are pointing to the possible decline in importance of the nation state arising from these processes of globalisation it has been a concomitant development that citizen rights and obligations may correspondingly be less strongly aligned on a national basis (Soysal, 1998). Instead, some have championed a 'cosmopolitan view that human well-being is not defined by geographical or cultural locations' (Held 2004: xi). The idea here is that, increasingly, citizenship rights and obligations are less dependent upon membership of a particular territorial and legal society. Many people, described as *denizens* by Tomas Hammer (1990), increasingly live and work in countries in which they were neither born nor naturalised. Thus it becomes possible for denizens to have different rights and obligations to a number of 'wider societies' and experience a series of transnational and transitional citizen statuses. Moreover, a range of transnational procedures and institutions have facilitated an increase in the cross-border flow of migrant denizens, which may reinforce such trends.

National identity, as a collection of symbols, values and practices which inform young people's sense of citizenship may therefore come to be regarded as one among a number of competing identities. These alternative sites for citizenship identity are further intensified for young people in many late modern societies by the advent of multiculturalism as a social characteristic. First and second generation immigrants may have less difficulty in identifying with both their countries of birth and those of cultural heritage. They might, for example, be members of the UK armed forces and supporters of the visiting Pakistani cricket team to England. Moreover, those who live in such multicultural societies are both subject to the cultural benefits such diversity brings as well as the social tensions which may arise. But the growing liquidity and mobility of large sections of populations (Urry, 2000; Bauman, 2005) exposes many younger people to a broader range of influences than previous generations. In, sometimes, stark contrast it also reveals new social divisions between those who experience greater mobility and those who are involuntarily embedded.

The weakening of national identity may further be associated with the perceived weakness of national politicians and institutions to deal effectively with many of the global political issues which concern young people. Environmental damage to the planet and poverty in the developing world, for example, consistently challenge traditional national attempts to deal with global commercial interests, transnational regulation and economic liberalisation. Such disenchantment with national politics may be further extended by government's failure to meet demands from rising welfare expectations. Kenneth Galbraith (1992) cogently outlined the challenge confronting late modern democratic welfare states as a 'culture of contentment'. While the majority of voters are increasingly well off and self-interested, they are content to use their electoral advantage to oppose public expenditure and state interference which might meet the needs of the socially and politically excluded. Increasingly bereft of the national security provided from welfare institutions, young people may be less likely therefore to develop that sense of social obligation which would underpin a commitment and identification with the welfare state exhibited by previous generations.

Deinstitutionalisation and social fragmentation

The social construction of political identity is further complicated for young people as a consequence of the sociological and cultural changes postulated in much contemporary social theory (Giddens, 1991; Castells, 2001; Lash, 2002; Urry, 2003; Bauman, 2005; Sennett, 2006). Despite the expected disagreement about the precise nature and future direction of the social and political development underway there does seem to be a consensus that late modern advanced societies are subject to significant institutional and cultural changes arising from an increasingly global informational economy (Castells, 1996). Traditional social and cultural institutions (families, voluntary organisations, churches, employment organisations), which provided collective political meaning, symbols and authority for young people are being challenged by processes of deinstitutionalisation (Bennett, 1998; Beck, 2000).

Related to the weakening sense of obligation to traditional social institutions has been a significant decline in the importance of *social class* as a signifier of political identity and allegiance. In many late modern societies, deindustrialisation, automation and a notable increase in white-collar employment has seen the working classes diminish both in size and political relevance. So here too we have another example of how the political socialisation and identity of working-class young people into the values of solidarity, trust and collective action, in relation to the 'wider society' is being eroded as a consequence of social restructuring and the accompanying decline of local communities. The old values, norms and affinities conforming with social class identity are being transformed and replaced with the prospect of multiple identities arising from new social distinctions such as gender, sexuality, race and disability, which confront young people in contemporary societies.

Individualisation and consumerism

Associated with these developments in social fragmentation has been a corresponding emphasis upon the individual and the process of self-reflexivity (Giddens, 1991). The disconnection with social class and political institutions identified above has led to a corresponding shift in social obligation and rights, such that individuals are being required to take more responsibility for managing their own lifestyle choices, risk assessments and life plans (Giddens, 1991; Beck, 1999; Bennett, 1998; Loader, 1998). There are many manifestations, but they encompass individualised agendas characterised by the ongoing activities of choosing between various lifestyle and fashion statements, shaping and expressing one's persona, celebrating body forms and artistry, and developing and managing social networks of friends, family and associates. Significantly, such social action increasingly takes place within a consumerist and lifestyle orientated context where the rights and obligations of citizens are much harder to discern. Instead, citizenship identity appears to be more closely associated with the development of individual preferences related to lifestyle and consumer politics. Unlike more stable forms of social class, religious or national political identities, these deinstitutionalised identities may take multiple forms and be transitory in nature.

Such developments pose serious problems for conventional political organisations to interpret changing public opinion or manage intelligible political mobilisation. Indeed, Pattie *et al.* (2004) hold the view that citizenship is still best understood in relation to geographical locality:

> Citizenship is more likely to emerge among equals in a permanently settled community who are neighbours and who have a forum in which they can interact and where the institution can impose sanctions . . . Nationalism is very helpful in supporting citizenship because it binds together people who are geographically separated, and who are never likely to meet each other face-to-face, into 'imaginary communities'.
>
> (2004: 21)

For them and those of similar persuasion, such bonds of social obligation and cultural identity cannot be achieved at the transnational level where neighbours are literally too far removed to illicit sacrifice or common understanding. Similarly, support for compulsory redistributive taxation is much harder to maintain without strong ties of social obligation based upon relatively homogeneous societies compared to larger heterogeneous ones (ibid.).

Civic participation and political activism

The debates over the normative dimensions of citizenship provide the context for the behavioural roles of citizens to solve collective action problems. Political participation and civic engagement are usually considered by means of a continuum (see Vromen, Chapter 7). At its most limited, the role of the citizen in a democratic society might require the voluntary action of voting which might expand into making donations, joining a political party, contacting officials and attending political meetings. Following on from their earlier definition, Pattie *et al.*, suggest that a good citizen 'would be someone who is aware of their rights, but also their obligations to other people and the wider society. In addition, good citizens participate in voluntary activities of various kinds as well as politics more generally . . .' (2004: 129).

It is precisely these forms of participation which the *disaffected citizen* proponents argue that young people are failing to adopt. They presumably can be considered to be closer to what Pattie *et al.*, regard as a 'bad citizen' concerned only to demand 'their rights, but . . . reluctant to acknowledge their obligations to the rest of society' (2004: 130). In the UK 2005 general election, for example, it was estimated that only 37 per cent of 18- to 24-year-olds voted (a decline from 39 per cent on 2001). Explanations for citizen disaffection come from assorted sources but a popular account was provided by Robert Putnam in his widely cited book *Bowling Alone* (2000). Putnam charts the growing apathy towards civic participation in American society where once the high levels of social support, voluntary activity and neighbourhood engagement were characterised by communities regularly going out and playing ten-pin bowling together. He amasses an impressive body of evidence in support of the view that where active civic engagement or 'social capital' is prevalent it has beneficial effects upon individual health, education, security and employment prospects. Interestingly, it is to the media that Putnam points the finger of accusation as the most significant cause for disaffection and breakdown of civic engagement. Instead of engaging in the public domain Americans have become spectators of the public sphere through the television in their private realm.

This explanation of the television as a reason for the rise of public disengagement with politics has been postulated by several commentators. Neil Postman and Jürgen Habermas, for example, both in their respective approaches argue that the televisual media have a negative impact upon the democratic sphere by privileging the visual image over text. The communication of print culture, Postman argued, was 'generally coherent, serious and rational' in contrast to television where 'it has become shrivelled and absurd' (1987: 16). Whereas previous generations were more likely to be literate, have long attention spans and be capable of following complex political discussions, television 'requires minimal skills to comprehend it, and it is aimed largely at emotional gratification' (ibid. 88–9). Habermas, in his earlier work, made similarly disparaging observations about 'the replacement of a reading public that debates critically about matters of culture by the mass public of culture consumers' (1989: 168). It is the technology of the printing press and the sustained engagement with reading that enabled the 'public' to criticise the government and hold their representatives accountable. Thus, it is primarily through reasoned deliberation and communication that civic engagement and participation are able to foster and enable democratic politics.

The now familiar arguments about political communication being 'dumbed down' on television would seem to bear testimony to Postman and Habermas's prognostications. The public are daily subjected to a schedule of political soundbites, party advertising, policy brands and celebrity images, which are aimed at the citizen consumers choosing their public services on the basis of commercial marketing techniques. As armies of communications consultants, designers and marketing analysts maintain a constant campaign to engineer public opinion for citizens in the comfort of their own homes the necessity to engage in public life becomes diminished. Moreover, citizens become less well equipped to challenge the truth or falsehood of mass mediated political discourse in any literate, analytical or reasoned way. Not only does this contribute to the disengagement of citizens from political participation but it also contributes to disaffection with political democracy by both increasing individual public service consumer demands, which cannot be met, as well as producing mistrust of political representatives.

The adherents of the *cultural displacement* perspective are both more cautious about the debilitating effects of mass media and also suggest that the new media of the Internet may offer wider opportunities for understanding political participation. In the first place by taking a broader view of political participation they look to the level of engagement through such activities as marching, protesting and striking as additional indicators of the strength of the democratic polity. Instead of focusing upon political consensus and agreement as the measure of democratic society, they would point to the value of conflict and opposition as a requirement for strong democracy (Mouffe, 1992). Thus challenging civil and democratic institutions, either through direct action or by withdrawing support, may also be considered to come within the remit of democratic politics. The rejection of arrogant and self-absorbed professional politics may not be a cynical withdrawal but rather interpreted as the beginnings of a legitimate opposition.

Second, the *cultural displacement* view is less pessimistic about the one-dimensional cultural hegemony of the mass media and suggests instead that the public are capable of both critically interpreting the marketing messages of politicians and retaining their own political views. Thus, instead of mediated popular youth culture being regarded as a domain of political control, it can rather be seen as a more complex environment where autonomy and agency can mobilise political action. The behavioural roles of youth citizens no longer need to be considered solely in relation to the state and representative politics but also through a variety of private and public activities from shopping to online global campaigning, culture jamming and cyberprotesting (Donk *et al.*, 2004), which reflect the concerns and processes of individualisation and deinstitutionalisation confronting young citizens.

New media, political socialisation and citizenship education

The potential of new media to regenerate democratic politics was eagerly championed by enthusiasts of digital democracy during the first wave of the Internet 'revolution' (Loader, 1997; Hague and Loader, 1999). The adoption of global, flexible computer network communications seemed to offer the prospect of an online Habermassian public sphere which was open to all the world's citizens to share information, engage in political deliberation and challenge state authority (Barlow, 1996a, 1996b). Despite the somewhat disappointing realisation of electronic democracy to date (Kamark and Nye, 2002) the appeal of new media as a means of socialising and mobilising young citizens remains strong. In contrast to earlier cyber-utopias contemporary techno-visions draw upon a mixture of the 'everyday lifeworld' of young Internet users and the cultural changes in late modern societies already discussed. They are based, no doubt, partly upon the experiential observations of young people celebrating their familiarity and playful enjoyment of the new media. But they also encompass an electoral affinity between the enthusiastic adoption of the new media by young people and the wider opportunities for political action around lifestyle and consumer politics discussed above, which resonate more with contemporary youth culture.

As a consequence, researchers have become interested in whether online interaction provides either alternative or complementary avenues for political socialisation. Within the *cultural displacement* framework these have focused upon both the role ICTs can play in citizenship education and also how political parties can design websites and develop an online presence attractive to young people. For the dislocated citizen perspective it manifests itself as a search for evidence of the Internet as an alternative sphere for mobilisation, which may be more cosmopolitan in style and content. Online activists, for example, have utilised sophisticated marketing techniques to design websites which challenge what they regard as unacceptable corporate practices disguised by well-known brands (Klein, 2000). Are such culture jamming websites more appealing as a means to engage young people in democratic action? Does contributing to online campaigns provide young people with citizen skills and political understanding that lead to further public participation? Does the online web sphere relate to the multiple identity and mobile nature of contemporary youth culture? Can such flexible online networking sustain the trust and commitment required for mobilisation?

Debating young citizens in the digital age

As outlined above the contributions to this collection address the tensions and themes which arise from the competing *citizen disaffection* and *cultural displacement* perspectives of young people's engagement and participation in democratic life. While the authors may not wish to be assigned to either position, the framework, nonetheless, provides a useful dialectic to foreground current arguments about the influence of new media for the political socialisation and engagement of young people in late modern democracies. The book is structured into two parts. In the first, we focus upon those analyses of how young people currently use the Internet. This is followed in Part II by a number of contributions related to strategies, pedagogies and campaigns to increase the political participation of young people through the new media.

Part I begins with a chapter by **Sonia Livingstone**, **Nick Couldry** and **Tim Markham** who provide an empirical analysis of young people's online activities drawing upon data from two UK projects that they have undertaken. Since one of these investigations samples adults the authors are able to assess the significance of any generational differences in online use. The authors explore the contention that the Internet has become a means of revitalising the democratic involvement of young people through the variety of projects and opportunities available online. Their findings strongly support the view that while online interactivity and creativity can be stimulated through the experience of using the Internet, the likelihood of civic engagement online is significantly influenced by offline demographic factors. Thus political mobilisation through the Internet appears to be limited by the extent of prior political interests and understanding. For those already imbued with civic awareness the Internet provides a useful resource for pursuing such interests but it does not in itself provide an inducement to political understanding and participation. Thus, young citizens cannot easily dislocate to alternative online political spaces without having first been socialised in their offline everyday lives.

These findings not only make a strong link between the online and offline demographic experiences of political socialisation but they also reaffirm young people's perceptions of democratic politics even when manifested online. The authors concur that young people are more interested in celebrity and related contemporary culture than current political offerings whether online or not. Thus, they are indeed disaffected with traditional politics but are as yet largely unimpressed by the Internet as a means to become more engaged. While acknowledging some indications of young people using the Internet to access civic, news and political sites, Livingstone and her colleagues could find little evidence for the Internet as a primary source of political socialisation compared with its value as a resource for leisure and social relations more generally.

Through an analysis of Internet usage for political purposes by young people during the 2005 UK general election, **Gustavo S. Mesch** and **Stephen Coleman** also provide support for the contention that offline socio-economic and gender differences in civic participation are largely replicated online. Again, this points to the role of the Internet for reinforcing existing democratic awareness rather than as an alternative mode of political socialisation. However, their findings were not wholly contrary to the *cultural displacement* hypothesis. Interestingly, as a percentage of the online population accessing political information during the campaign, young people were much more likely to use the Internet for news-related websites and information about candidates and parties than were older users. This suggests that online strategies by political parties to target young voters were a valuable approach in attracting disaffected young citizens. However, it also indicates that political engagement by young people may show signs of becoming dislocated to the new media where mobilisation and activism may be more heightened if they are Internet users.

So too an analysis of the 2004 USA presidential election campaign by **Michael Xenos** and **W. Lance Bennett** provides a mixed set of results for the promises and potentialities of the Internet as a conduit for engaging young citizens. In this case the election witnessed a dramatic reversal of the disaffection trend with an increase in youth participation and engagement. This surge was interpreted by some commentators as a vindication of the adoption of new media by the campaign teams and candidates to capture the youth vote. In their interpretation, however, Xenos and Bennett suggest that this 'technological fix' disguises the influence of the intense offline canvassing and get-the-vote efforts directed at young people. Thus, while the rise in political interest among young citizens may have been partly due to enhanced Internet sites and more sophisticated online campaigning, many other factors unrelated to online politics also made a contribution.

From the perspective of the dislocated young citizen hypothesis, Xenos and Bennett also provide some interesting findings. Described as the *youth political web sphere*, the authors explored a collection of sites which were designed to interest young people in politics generally that were not sponsored by any official parties or candidates. Here their analysis reveals some promising opportunities for mobilising young people through the visual and interactive features of sites that are more familiar to their experience. These contrasted markedly with the campaign and candidate web sphere, which may crucially limit the extent of connectivity between the two political web spheres.

If we move away from the idea of the Internet as some kind of alternative space, unrelated to the offline world, which can act to politically socialise young people independently of more traditional socio-demographic factors, and instead consider its impact on those already politically engaged, do we get a different picture of young people mobilised online? **Peter Dahlgren** and **Tobias Olsson**, in Chapter 5, report on a qualitative research project which interviewed young people who were politically active in either traditional political parties or alternative 'new' political groups. They argue for a more contextualised view of the Internet as one of a number of media in young people's lives in order to assess its importance relative to other sources of influence.

The analytical frame for the investigation adopted by Dahlgren and Olsson is fashioned by concepts of civic identity and practices associated with late modern society. Thus, their findings are important as a means of gauging the cogency of the *cultural displacement* hypothesis. Is the Internet responsible for developing the civic identity of young people engaged in 'new' social movements or other extra-parliamentary politics? Once again, the argument is strongly made that the Internet does not provide a separate sphere for the construction of an online civic identity. Rather, the Internet is an important medium for making a significant contribution to the multifaceted ongoing development of existing (mainly offline) identity construction.

For those young people actively engaged in new political movements and networks, the value of the Internet is clearly evidenced. Dahlgren and Olsson report on several examples of the creative and innovative use of the new media by young citizens. The additional advantages of the Internet over traditional media were expressed by the respondents who cited its value for alternative sources of information, internal coordination, mobilisation and access to public spheres. Consequently, the Internet can be seen as an important resource, together with other media, for the processes of dislocation which may be exhibited by those young citizen activists.

In Italy, a familiar picture of young people distrusting their politicians is outlined by **Davide Calenda** and **Lorenzo Mosca** but this is paradoxically combined with a strong politicisation of young people compared with older generations. This underlying trend reveals a favouritism for progressive and left-leaning politics within this group and again may suggest evidence for the argument that young people are positive about politics and civic engagement but not with the style or format in which it is currently being provided. Drawing upon data arising from two surveys of Italian students, Calenda and Mosca attempt to establish whether and how the political characteristics of this sample influence the way in which they use the Internet for political activity.

Their analysis identified two important relationships between online and offline participation which concur with many of the empirical investigations considered in this collection. First, the authors also confirm that the Internet is perceived and utilised as a valuable resource for those young students already politically engaged offline. Second, the findings do not reveal significant differences in the style of political participation between online and offline activities. Instead, the Internet typically provides a bridge for these interviewees between offline ties and associations and the continued debate and non face-to-face interaction.

A further international comparison of young people's use of the Internet for political participation is provided by **Ariadne Vromen** whose Australian survey demonstrates that a socio-democratic digital divide is a prominent factor influencing engagement. The quantitative evidence provided by two case studies of non-government organisations that use the Internet to facilitate participation are also instructive of the value of youth-led political spaces for political engagement. But once again it is offline political socialisation and a variety of other media sources, such as television and newspapers, which influences the use of the Internet for young people's engagement rather than the obverse.

Vromen, like previous contributors, does not detect any significant difference in the form of participation online. Is this a consequence, in part, of the methodology adopted to analyse online behaviour? **Roman Gerodimos** and **Janelle Ward** take a critical look at web content analysis which has been influential as a method of researching online political communication. Their contention is that traditional offline approaches to content analysis should not simply be transplanted to online communication. Instead, they argue that changes in content, space, time and the reach of young people's online political communication requires new methods and techniques. As a way forward they consider triangulating content analysis with other methods, which they outline for consideration.

In Part II of this collection we turn our attention to how the affinity of young people with new media has been as an important driver for the contribution of ICTs for contemporary political socialisation. The remaining five chapters together provide a picture, albeit partial rather than comprehensive, of the UK's experience of a mixture of policies, institutions and initiatives specifically designed to incorporate new media in order to engage young people in civic participation. The British Government's response to the disaffection of young people with democratic politics was to make citizenship education compulsory in schools as a part of the national curriculum. **Neil Selwyn** in Chapter 9 documents the inappropriate use of ICTs to date in the national curriculum as a technological fix to what I have called the *disaffected citizen* problem. Instead, Selwyn suggests that ICT-based citizenship education would be more in tune with the online experience of young people if it were more personalised and focused around lifestyle politics. Moreover, he is at pains to point out that citizenship education cannot simply be the responsibility of schools and teachers alone. The wider community of stakeholders such as family, politicians, religious and civic leaders all have their part to play.

A range of online tools for citizenship education has been provided by the Hansard Society's *HeadsUp* project which is explained by its director **Ross Ferguson**. The experimental initiative provides as its centrepiece an online deliberative forum. Topics suggested by the young people are debated with the participation of parliamentarians, schools and prospective young citizens. Again, the tentative results suggest an important online tool for connecting a range of stakeholders involved in citizenship education and the potential for greater efficacy through politicians learning directly about the concerns and views of young people.

The importance of deliberation for democratic citizenship is further explored in a case study by **Roger Austin**, who examines the potential value and challenges of using ICT to enable a divided society to work together. In Northern Ireland religious factionalism and related separate faith schooling provide the context for an online pilot designed to facilitate the intercultural understanding necessary for reconnecting young people to each other as a platform for wider political deliberation. In this instance, it is not the content of democratic citizenship which is foregrounded but rather the structured use of ICTs to facilitate collaborative work across the divide, which opens up the possibility for respecting differences and celebrating diversity.

The collection concludes with a robust proposition by **Stephen Coleman** that it is formal democratic politics which has become disconnected with contemporary youth culture rather than that young people have become disaffected with politics. And this needs to be acknowledged. He maintains that the language and style of politicians fails to address the values, experiences and concerns of young people. Instead, political elites need to recognise that political culture has to change in line with wider popular culture if it is to attract the interest of younger people. TV reality shows like *Big Brother*, and interactive new media, argues Coleman, may provide more instructive pointers for politicians to reconnect with young people than a stubborn retention of outmoded audience reception models of political communication.

Concluding remark

In summary, the contributions to this collection provide an international range of empirical data from which to analyse the adoption of new media by young people and ascertain the influence it has upon their political participation in late modern societies. It also documents a number of initiatives designed to engage young people in democratic politics. The analyses have been undertaken within the context of the current debate, which we have characterised as comprising a distinction between those social theorists adopting a *disaffected young citizen* perspective and those who can be more associated with a *cultural displacement* approach.

As might be expected, the results are somewhat mixed and do not allow for one approach to be completely privileged over the other. It can be said, however, that the contributions provide strong support for the role of new media in young people's lives and a reaffirmation of the negative view of politics held by young people. Yet it is important that the value of the Internet for political socialisation should not be exaggerated and regarded as separated from offline influences (including traditional media) and socio-demographic characteristics which continue to be paramount. But evidence is also provided which suggests that new media could be positive in its impact where young people are already politically active. Although the gap between the youth political web sphere and the formal political campaigning sphere appears to be large in the view of young online activists it remains to be seen if links will be made between them in the future. What then becomes interesting is how new media might interact not to form a new media age replete with entirely new political cultures but rather to contribute to existing trends towards individualised, celebrity, consumerist and aethetised politics.

Any attempts, therefore, to reconnect with young people would appear to require democratic institutions and practices to restyle their political communication in such ways as to be commensurate with the interests and discourse of contemporary youth culture in an increasingly deinstitution-alised and personalised social world. As the generation whose lifestyle most encompasses the use of digital communications it should be no surprise that the creative adoption of new media, such as the Internet, to engage young citizens would be an essential element of this restyling strategy. But it also necessitates an acknowledgement of the wider changing social conditions and political culture within which young people must now operate and how this relationship is mediated by ICTs. Young people are not alone as an age group in disconnecting from the traditional institutions, symbols and authorities that shaped political meaning, identification and action in many twentieth-century democratic nation states. They are, rather, the most statistically significant example of such recent trends and are the first to experience the late modern social condition arising from global production, communication and consumption.

Part I
Young citizens online

2 Youthful steps towards civic participation

Does the Internet help?

Sonia Livingstone, Nick Couldry and Tim Markham

Declining participation offline, rising participation online

Our recent Public Connection Survey, which surveyed 1,017 people aged 18+ across the UK in June 2005, found that young people (18–34) are less likely to vote in national elections, compared with middle-aged (35–54) and older (55+) people (Couldry *et al.*, 2006). Indeed, 89 per cent of over 55s, but only 67 per cent of under 35s, said they 'generally vote in national elections'.[1] Similarly, 75 per cent of over 55s claimed to be 'generally interested in what's going on in politics', compared with only 61 per cent of under 35-year-olds. Yet, the survey also found, as have many others, that young people are much more likely to use the Internet. Almost no teenagers in the UK are non-users (just 2–3 per cent; Livingstone and Helsper, in press), 72 per cent of 18–35s go online daily, while 75 per cent of over 55s do not use it at all. Putting together the declining vote and political interest among young adults with the distinctively youthful profile of Internet users, one would hardly suppose that the Internet could be part of the solution to the decline in political participation among young people. Indeed, it seems more likely to be part of the problem – an update, perhaps, on Putnam's (2000) *Bowling Alone* thesis, in which the Internet, rather than television, serves to fragment and distract a youthful public from a common sense of civic purpose.[2]

Nonetheless, a growing body of research and, especially, policy hopes to invert this pessimistic conclusion, seeking to capitalise on young people's interest in the Internet to encourage them into a greater engagement with politics (Center For Media Education, 2002; Levine and Lopez, 2004; Lusoli *et al.*, 2006; Newman *et al.*, 2004). After all, young people undoubtedly use the Internet to sustain and extend their communication networks, and they commit to these networks a considerable investment in time, motivation, sociability and identity. In the UK Children Go Online (UKCGO) project, which surveyed 1,511 9- to 19-year-olds, children and teenagers were found to spend, on average, between half an hour and one hour per day online,[3] a little more than the half-hour per day average spent by the

18- to 34-year-olds surveyed in the Public Connection project, and much more than for older groups (less than 15 minutes for those aged 55+).[4]

In short, young people are generally enthusiastic and creative adopters of the Internet – especially for communication, information, entertainment and education, enjoying their expertise in using the Internet, notwithstanding some limits to these skills particularly in critical and productive literacies (Livingstone, 2007). Thus, they are constantly connected (Clark, 2005) being, as Subrahmanyam *et al.*, (2001) argue, primarily social rather than anti-social, oriented towards constructing community, albeit a community that sustains and prioritises their interests and in which they have a stake. But one must remain cautious as to whether these networked weak ties (Hampton and Wellman, 2003) truly merit the label of 'community', for it is unclear that such connection leads them to political or civic engagement, either on or offline.

In this chapter, we draw together the findings of two projects, one on teens, one on adults, which have been conducted separately but with overlapping theoretical frameworks and methods, in order to generate a picture of young people's sense of 'public connection'[5] as they make the transition from adolescence to young adulthood.[6] Although we cannot here disentangle the effects of generational change from life course transitions, these projects do allow us to address the common problem that, first, surveys of political participation (and of media/technology use) typically survey only adults, impeding a view of the transition to adulthood (or, problematically, relying on adult, that is, parental, accounts of young people's media or social activities); second, surveys of young people are frequently interpreted as revealing findings distinctive to young people, without realising that, had an older sample been included, similar findings would apply across the age range.

For example, in both projects, respondents were asked whether they go online for news. Among the UKCGO sample, 17 per cent of 12- to 15-year-olds claim to do this, compared with 34 per cent of 16- to 17-year-olds and 41 per cent of 18- to 19-year-olds. Asked the slightly different question of whether they go online to read the news at least three times per week, the Public Connection Survey found 40 per cent of 18- to 35-year-olds do this, compared with 25 per cent of 35- to 54-year-olds and only 7 per cent of over 55s. There is, in short, a peak between 18 and 35, with younger and older age groups being less likely to seek their news online. Without the Public Connection data, one might suppose that teenagers differ from all adults; without the UKCGO data, one would not know how online news consumption jumps in mid to late adolescence and, perhaps, assume it to be typical of all younger members of 'the Internet generation'.

Contextualising online news in a broader perspective reveals further that, even for young adults who get news online, longer-established media remain a more important news source, with 54 per cent of 18 to 35-year-olds reading a national paper at least three times per week, 70 per cent listening to the radio news and 87 per cent watching television news – all figures not very different from those for older age groups. Young people's consumption of Internet news is, undoubtedly, distinctive – but it should also be recognised that the Internet supplements rather than displaces other news sources (Althaus and Tewksbury, 2000),[7] and television remains 'the main source' (Robinson and Levy, 1986). If we exclude interpersonal media (the mobile phone), television remains the medium that would be most missed by 16–24 year olds, just as for older ages (Ofcom, 2006: 74). Moreover, although young people draw on a more diverse news environment than older generations, young people's interest in the Internet is insufficient to counter their generally lower levels of news consumption overall (Pew, 2002, 2004b, 2005). Thus, the Internet remains less important as a primary news source than recent hype about the Internet replacing television consumption would suggest, leading us to disagree, at least at present, with Haythornthwaite and Wellman (2002): in the UK at least, 'the person' – even the young person – has *not* become 'the portal' to public information flows.

Online invitations to participate

According to the producers of civic websites for youth, many young people are eagerly and creatively engaging with the online invitation to join in, to have their say, to represent themselves (Livingstone, in press-a). Young people, they claim, have a right to express themselves, for their voices to become visible, and the online community is keen for their contribution: allowing young people to 'be heard' is a common feature of the design characteristics and interface of youth civic websites. Indeed, the promise of youth websites is built on the supposed parallels between young people's preferred style of interaction (dialogic, diverse, alternative, dynamic) and the infrastructure of the Internet (peer-to-peer, heterogenous, flexible). More generally, governments appear optimistic that civic or political participation can be revitalised by involving the Internet, thus initiating a range of projects for cultural citizenship, political socialisation, participatory deliberation, e-democracy, and so forth (Bentivegna, 2002; Coleman, 2005a; Livingstone, 2005).[8]

Such optimism is not always borne out in practice. The UKCGO project asked, as one strand of the research, whether taking up the 'invitation' to interact online – completing quizzes, voting on entertainment websites, contributing to message boards, and so forth – does, in fact, lead young people (here, teenagers aged 12–17) into an online engagement with civic or political sites (Livingstone *et al.*, 2005). Looking across the various forms of participation online, the UKCGO project found that most activities are positively, if weakly, correlated among young people (in other words, the more young people use the Internet for any one activity, the more they use it for the others, and vice versa), suggesting a positive transfer of skills and interests across online activities, including the possibility that young people who engage with the interactive potential of the Internet become drawn into a civic participation. However, although use of email and information search is widespread, levels of news-seeking and advice-seeking (along with the use of the Internet to mediate club-related or other organised social activities) are all rather low, pursued by around a quarter of young Internet users, and are often short-lived, indicating difficulties with 'following through' rather than with initial enthusiasm. Possibly, the forms of interacting with websites that are practiced fairly commonly (for example, completing quizzes, sending emails) may already be familiar practices offline (for example, quizzes in magazines, phoning a radio programme). Less common practices online may reflect the fact that young people are not used to receiving and responding to requests to vote, offer advice, sign a petition and so forth in their everyday (offline) lives.

Of greater concern is the fact that online opportunities are not taken up equally. Not only do boys, middle-class and older teens have higher levels of Internet self-efficacy, stay online longer per day and have longer experience with the Internet, but these factors – both demographic and use-related – seem to facilitate the take-up of online opportunities to interact. In other words, it appears that online interactivity and creativity can be encouraged through the very experience of using the Internet. However, this is less the case for the likelihood of visiting civic websites because here the key determinants are demographic – age (older), gender (girls) and social class (higher). This suggests that young people's motivation to pursue civic interests online depends on their background and their socialisation, and it is not greatly affected by the amounts of time spent or levels of expertise online. Rather, those with prior civic or political interests find the Internet a useful resource for pursuing these interests; similarly, those motivated to explore the Internet creatively do so, resulting in an active and creative engagement with the medium, but not necessarily drawing them into greater civic or political engagement than before. In short, interaction and civic engagement are not to be regarded as sequenced 'steps' on a 'ladder' of participation from minimal to more ambitious modes of participation (Hill and Tisdall, 1997).

Rather than blaming young people for their apathy, the finger might instead be pointed at the online and offline structures of opportunity that facilitate, shape and develop young people's participation. Focus groups with young people suggest a generation bored with politics, critical of the online offer, instead interested in celebrity and conforming to peer norms (Livingstone, in press-a). Young people protest that 'having your say' does not seem to mean 'being listened to', and so they feel justified in recognising little responsibility to participate (Lister *et al.*, 2003). In this respect, they resemble the general UK population (Power, 2006). Indeed, evaluations of some online initiatives are less than optimistic (Liff *et al.*, 2002; Phipps, 2000): an American survey of 15- to 25-year-olds found the Internet an even less effective means of engaging disaffected young people than traditional routes, though very effective at mobilising the already-interested (Levine and Lopez, 2004; see also Livingstone, *et al.*, 2005). Young people are often positioned by even the most well-meaning public sector sites not as citizens but as citizens-in-waiting (Buckingham, 2000; Qvortrup, 1995) and, it seems that while they wait to become fully fledged citizens, young people can think of better things to do with their time. Thus, one is tempted to suggest that it is those making the invitation, not those responding to it, that lack the motivation to participate in a dialogue with young people. Cammaerts and Van Audenhove (2005) show how online discussions reveal a series of constraints that undermine the freedom of the so-called public sphere online, while Bessant (2004) notes, pessimistically, that despite the many calls to empower young people through the Internet, policy makers' enthusiasm tends to ignore the obstacles that youth experiences to participation socially, economically and politically, particularly the question of whose voice is being heard and to what effect.

Disconnected youth?

What, then, is distinctive about younger people as regards civic engagement? As Table 2.1 shows, they claim less interest in politics than do older people. But this is not, apparently, because they are *less* trusting of politics (Aday, 2005), nor because they are lower on political efficacy (Inglehart, 1977). Young people are, undoubtedly, fairly low on both measures, but they are not significantly lower than the rest of the population.

The indicators that are significantly different by age are telling: young people are lower on social capital (Table 2.1; see also Field, 2003) and social expectations to 'keep up with what's going on in the world'. Further, young people's sense of what is going on in the world, the public (or new) agenda, is also distinctive. When asked which, if any, of a diverse list of eighteen items, 'do you generally follow or keep up to date with?' young people were significantly less likely than older people to select items concerned with traditional politics (such as 'trade union politics', 'international politics', 'what's happening in Iraq', 'the UK economy', 'local council politics', 'events in Westminster', 'funding for local services', 'debates about Europe'). They were also, perhaps more surprisingly, significantly less likely than older people to follow such single issues as 'health', 'crime', 'the environment' and 'third world poverty'. Last but not least, they were significantly more likely than older people to follow popular or celebrity issues: 'what's number one in the music charts', 'the latest celebrity gossip', 'the latest fashion in clothes', 'Big Brother or other reality television'. Note, finally, that as for political trust, young people are no more or less trusting of media sources, despite their greater propensity to keep up with celebrity

Table 2.1 Indicators of civic/political engagement, by age

	Age						Age difference?
	18–24	*25–34*	*35–44*	*45–54*	*55–64*	*65+*	
Civic/political engagement							
Political interest[9]	3.34	3.44	3.31	3.44	3.91	3.88	$p < 0.01$
Political trust[10]	2.79	2.60	2.75	2.60	2.67	2.69	n.s.
Political efficacy[11]	3.16	3.25	3.21	3.25	3.25	3.00	n.s.
Social capital[12]	2.72	2.57	2.73	2.80	2.97	2.87	$p < 0.01$
Social expectations[13]	3.06	3.31	3.48	3.52	3.70	3.62	$p < 0.01$
Media trust[14]	3.20	3.20	3.29	3.25	3.29	3.31	n.s.
Media literacy[15]	3.45	3.58	3.56	3.64	3.65	3.69	$p < 0.05$

Note: *Public Connection Survey* (2005) of British adults aged 18+ (N = 1007). See Couldry *et al.* (2006, in press-a). All indicators measured on a 5-point Likert-type scale from 1 = strongly disagree to 5 = strongly agree.

news. But they are rather less media literate – an intriguing finding given their more diverse media environment, offline and online.

The Public Connection project used these indicators to examine who goes online to read the news, looking across the adult population (N = 1017). A binomial regression analysis found age to be the key predictor (beta = − 0.314, p < 0.01). However, other variables added to the explanation: people of higher socioeconomic status (beta = 0.123, p < 0.01), men (beta = 0.062, p < 0.05), those interested in 'traditional' political issues (beta = 0.073, p < 0.05), those who feel a social expectation on them to 'keep up' with the news (beta = 0.071, p < 0.05) and those who consider that they know where to get the information they need (0.067, p < 0.05) are all more likely to go online for news at least three times per week (R-squared = 14.9 per cent).

This analysis suggests that, rather than the Internet encouraging political interest,[16] the Internet instead provides a route to pursue already existing civic interests. And these already existing interests, it seems, may derive from social capital and social expectations – in short, from opportunity structures of people's everyday lives. Thus, we require a structural account of the conditions of participation, the opportunity structures of the state, work, commerce, school, community and family, within which young people may exercise their agency (Livingstone, 2006; Meyer and Staggenborg, 1996; Pattie *et al.*, 2004).

Offline structures of disconnection and exclusion

Few young people today are entirely excluded from Internet use by lack of access, though lack of home access remains an issue for a substantial minority of children and teens (Livingstone and Helsper, in press). Website design, increasingly mirroring the 'look and feel' of commercial sites, has considerably improved the interactive potential of many civic and political sites though problems remain in supporting genuine interactivity (Livingstone, 2007). Since, however, young people's use of the Internet has increased far more rapidly than their use of the Internet for *civic* purposes, we must look to other explanations for disengagement. Guided by accounts of late modernity developed by Giddens, Beck and others, Bennett (1998) points to a third cause to account for both growing individualisation and declining political engagement among youth, namely the dramatic shifts in the labour market and the economy in the post-war period. He argues that what is 'replacing traditional civil society is a less conformist social world ... characterised by the rise of networks, issue associations, and lifestyle coalitions facilitated by the revolution in personalised, point-to-point communication' (p. 745). Thus 'personal and local' concerns increasingly dominate over 'national and governmental' concerns (p. 748).

Young people are surely in the vanguard here, being both enthusiasts for individualised consumption but also struggling with the loss of clear structures of involvement and participation (the loss of jobs-for-life and clear employment trajectories, diminished local political organisations or trade unions, and increased economic pressures and debts) (Hill and Tisdall, 1997; James *et al.*, 1998). Not only do institutional structures present a stratified array of opportunities and constraints largely beyond young people's control but traditional cues to participation and citizenship are diminishing (Kimberlee, 2002; Touraine, 2000) as the commodification of childhood and youth increases (James *et al.*, 1998; Livingstone, 2002). Moreover, despite widespread optimism regarding online youth participation, and 'despite the recognition of children as persons in their own right, public policy and practice is marked by an intensification of control, regulation and surveillance around children, this impeding rather than facilitating the ability of organisations to encourage children's participation' (Prout, 2000), not least because 'children's participation can threaten adult hegemony and established practice' (Hill and Tisdall, 1997: 36).

In short, the (problematic) online opportunity structure available to young people may be no better than that established offline. Two of the younger participants in the Public Connection project (Jonathan and Josh, both aged 23) complained that they had no one offline with whom to discuss politics and public affairs, but interestingly, although both were active Internet users, neither mentioned online networks as compensating for this offline lack. We suggest, then, that it is the institutional structures (school, family, peers) that shape young people's daily lives and enable young people to engage with the civic or public sphere, whether on or offline, though the evidence regarding the social and political preconditions for young people's civic engagement (where it exists) remains unclear.

Test case studies – Anisah and Mary

During the course of these research projects, we visited a range of people at home – people of all ages and diverse backgrounds. In this section, we present just two case studies. These were selected not for their typicality, although they are in many ways ordinary young women, but because they illustrate the, as yet, tenuous links between daily life, civic commitments and Internet use. Indeed, while the UKCGO project showed how, for many, an enthusiastic and regular engagement with the Internet did not necessarily direct young people into online civic engagement, the Public Connection project found that for most people, young and old, there are only limited signs that Internet news consumption is generating sufficiently stable habits to replace the established domestic and cultural traditions of television news viewing or newspaper reading that mediates people's sense of public connection.

Anisah[17] is from a low-income Ghanaian family living on a troubled inner-city housing estate. The first author visited her initially when she was 12, in 1999, when the family lived in a very small two-bedroom flat, the computer being squeezed into the living room along with most other family activities. Her well-educated parents have placed huge educational expectations on their children, and so sought to provide the best for them, including several sets of encyclopaedias and educational CD-ROMs, a personal computer and Internet access. An active and outgoing girl, Anisah nonetheless lived far from her school friends and so spent a fair amount of time on her own. She used the Internet on most days, finding it exciting to make friends in chat rooms, and enjoying feeling ahead of her classmates in having domestic Internet access with which to research school projects. The Internet, she said, is better than books – quicker and more precise – though her skills are imperfect: she told us about a school project on China (the country) for which she downloaded an illustration of china (porcelain, in this case from America). By 2003, when we visited again, Anisah at 15 had become a charming and articulate teenager, doing well at school and hoping to become a designer. Having moved to a new house, she and her sister now have a bedroom to themselves and, to her delight, this also houses the computer. The Internet has become, for her, a key means of keeping in contact with the friends she sees every day at school, and she chats with them late into the night. Being about to enter her GSCE year, she also revises on the BBC's revision site, *Bitesize*, which she considers extremely helpful.

In terms of civic participation, Anisah's approach to life, including the Internet, has been strongly marked by her family's religious commitment, though she has become somewhat disengaged from the church, its legacy being her striking seriousness and moral conviction. Interestingly, she is the first and only child we have observed to read the news on the homepage of her Internet service provider – for although many enter through a page that contains headlines or direct links to the news, most pay no attention to this, going straight to their preferred links (email, entertainment, games, etc.). She has, further, become scathing of her earlier use of chat rooms, seeing this as a pointless, and possibly risky, waste of time. (Similarly, a young working-class participant in the Public Connection project – Kylie, 24 – dismissed Internet discussion: 'you're talking to people that are so far away from you'; Couldry *et al.*, 2007b). We also had an interesting discussion about how she, unlike her peers, refuses to download music, it being – she points out – both illegal and wrong. Thus she uses the Internet in a purposeful manner – to research artwork for a project, to follow her interest in design, to find a cheap flight, etc., relying largely but not solely on public-service oriented sites rather than commercial sites. And she told us how her father, similarly, reads the news online, particularly in order to follow the 'news and politics and what's happening' in Ghana. In short, Anisah illustrates the importance of family background – in terms of values and commitments, as well as Internet-related provision and practice – in shaping the way in which a young person uses the Internet for civic (and other) purposes. It is evident, nonetheless, that such civic purposes are not strong even for Anisah, that her use is fairly individualistic and strongly instrumental, and there is little evidence that she follows up on, or is drawn into, further civic engagement, having read the news or entered an educational site. Why then would one expect a less serious, less motivated or more fun-loving young person to see the Internet as a route to political engagement?

Mary's use of the Internet illustrates a further theme, reinforcing the importance of family background but adding to this the changing opportunity structures involved in the shift from adolescence to adulthood. Mary was 18 when we first visited, a school pupil finishing A levels, living in a well-off family in the rural north of England and hoping to study medicine. Like Anisah, she is ambitious, with a supportive family. Having reached voting age, she is well aware of her civic duty, but finds meeting this responsibility a challenge: 'I know what I'm thinking but I can't get it out properly . . . I can't put it into a proper argument.' Like Anisah too, she is instrumental in her information seeking, following up news or features on medicine, science, psychology and health, typically on television or in the press (we discuss designer babies, childhood obesity, cloning, etc.). Otherwise, she too fills the gaps between her studies by socialising with friends or watching 'rubbish on television'. Interestingly, her mother socialised her into reading the newspaper (the *Daily Mail*) quite deliberately: 'Mum always said I should look, she used to pick bits out for me to read, but then I suppose I just started doing it myself and I read more.' Similarly, she will watch the news headlines when the family is having their evening meal, because it is on, because her parents are watching it and because she can ask them (usually her mother) to explain the news to her. In addition to her family (including her argumentative father, with whom she tries not very successfully to test out her fledgling opinions), her school also provides a support structure that encourages engagement: she is a member of the school council, and this requires her to campaign for her own election, mentor junior pupils and 'do speeches and stuff'.

Yet the wider world of politics is something she has little interest in. She is happy to ask her parents' advice on how to vote, not always listening when they discuss politics at dinner, and expressing a mild scepticism of democratic participation ('Yeah, you're allowed to say what you think but it might not always be heard', she tells me – a view echoed by many young people). The Internet – crucially – plays a far lesser role in Mary's political socialisation or civic information seeking than does the everyday domestic context of family discussion and communal television news viewing. In the first interview, she told us about her family, school and social life, including her taste in television, magazines and radio, all before mentioning the Internet, which we had to introduce into the conversation. Then she said, 'I go on MSN and talk to my friends. . . . I use it for school work. . . . I just use it for work, all search engines and stuff.' Her account of learning to use the Internet differs strikingly from that of learning to read the newspapers: 'When we got it here, I started playing around and then I understood how to use it' – a free style of skill acquisition often described by young people, but one lacking in the social context that might direct them towards civic or political engagement. We asked whether she would look online to follow up something she's interested in from the world of science or medicine even, but she replied, 'I wouldn't look on the Internet. I would probably ask my Mum if there's anything in the paper about it or I'd have a look in the paper and then I'd sort of have a discussion with my Mum or Dad, Mum and Dad if, 'cos they'll, one of them will have heard about it.' When pushed about her information search, she said that for technical matters, she would ask a teacher instead, but the Internet is not, even for this educated and fairly privileged young woman, a main source.

On our follow-up visit, about six months later, Mary, a young adult of 19, was studying medicine at the local university. Her life on campus, in a shared student flat, was very different, and she had become far more confident and lively than the rather shy and uncertain person we met a few months earlier. She was working hard and playing hard, and though she saw her family, she had loosened the ties considerably (saying of her father, 'Well, he doesn't know what I'm doing now!'). Her media habits had changed dramatically – she no longer read the newspaper, didn't watch television ('I'm just hearing about things from word of mouth – I'm completely out of touch') and was about to get her own laptop with broadband Internet access. Two months later, in a focus group, she told the same story from a different perspective, having now returned home for the Christmas holiday: 'I . . . sort of got back into the news and knew what was going on again but all I know [normally at university] is the occasional bit I hear on the radio or what other people tell me.' The Internet clearly did not work to fill the gap. In the second interview she conceded, however, 'If I was desperate to know something, I'd sort of type in "news" in Google or something, don't know', though such desperation seems unlikely to her. However, she told us that in the intervening period between interviews, she did indeed vote, for the first time, in a recent local election, supporting the party favoured by her mother (less because of the issues than because, as her mother told her, women had to fight for the vote and so now they must use it). Again, we see the civic commitment of the parents continued in the children, yet Mary's confusion about politics remains: 'I suppose I'm not sure about the left and right wing really. I get confused with all the terms.' However, when asked if she had become involved in organisations at university, she described – with articulate confidence – her hopes of joining the medical students' society, the issues at stake and the processes involved. As before, the wider world of politics remained hazy (the news at the time of the interview was full of the 2005 American election, but she could not identify either candidates or issues involved), but the immediate world of her university, and her specialism, was vivid and engaging. The Internet, however, played little role in either.

Of course there are counter examples, cases of young people for whom the Internet is an important source of connection and participation (see Olsson, 2005a). Equally, there are many young people who lack the civic interest, family support, educational opportunities and/or the resources that both Anisah and Mary enjoy. Our point here is that, even with the civic interest, the family support, the educational opportunities and the resources to pursue their sense of public connection and civic engagement online, Anisah and Mary do not do so to any very great extent. Simply providing Internet access, or developing ever more well-meaning civic websites, is hardly going to be sufficient for the disengaged, disillusioned or disadvantaged, if this does not even succeed in engaging Anisah and Mary.

Conclusions

Many are asking whether the Internet affords new and emancipatory possibilities to inform and engage people. Others are critical of the 'techno-enthusiasm' (Selwyn, 2004) or 'cyberbole' (Woolgar, 2002) that has accompanied its arrival into the mass market, insisting on 'the contradiction between a for-profit, highly concentrated, advertising-saturated, corporate media system and the communication requirements of a democratic society' (McChesney, 2000, preface). Not only is it the case that 'the deployment of new technologies is always biased in some way to favour certain economic or social interests over others' (Mansell, 2004: 180), but also, as Graber (2004) rather reluctantly concludes, 'the Internet reinforces existing trends. It may be more than a blip, but it falls far short of being a revolution'. Winston (1996: 321), similarly, argues against the 'quite extraordinary claims' frequently made for the Internet, observing that the history of technology reveals that 'most such technologies exhibit far less radical potential'. Fornäs *et al.* (2002) comment more neutrally that new media may offer both reactionary as well as transformative possibilities, but point out that the structures of the offline world shape these possibilities such that 'tenacious structures in media institutions as well as in everyday-life contexts of use and production work to delimit the transformations first promised by each new medium, reproducing instead certain inherited boundaries in the new media as well'.

This chapter has argued more on the side of the pessimists rather than the optimists (Livingstone, 2005), not because the Internet is evidently undermining young people's participation, although the predominance of commercial rather than public sector content rightly gives cause for concern (Montgomery, 2001), nor because of the persistent inequalities in cultural and economic capital that shapes who gets access to the Internet (though this too is important), but rather because the Internet just does not yet show up as very important in relation to most young people's civic and political engagement, crucial though it is in many other domains of their life, such as, education, social relations, entertainment. Undoubtedly, some young people do engage effectively with the civic/public sphere, including via the Internet. Optimistic signs include the finding that young people are more likely to participate online than take part in more traditional forms of politics (Gibson *et al.*, 2002): while only 10 per cent of 15- to 24-year-olds in the UK took part in any form of political activity offline, three times that many did something political on the Internet. In the USA too, 38 per cent of 12- to 17-year-olds said they go online to express their opinion (Pew, 2001), and 26 per cent of the UKGCO teenagers go online to read the news. The lower commitment required for online participation, compared with attending meetings or other offline activities, may yet encourage young people. As Poppy (16, from London), reported: 'There's a Greenpeace website which had a petition about like global warming and stuff and we should do something about it. And I signed that just because it's easy and you might as well put your name down' (Livingstone, in press-b).

However, there is little evidence as yet that these young people are new to participation, or that the Internet draws in those not already engaged (Levine and Lopez, 2004; Livingstone, 2005; Olsson, 2005a) – the Internet is not, yet, 'the answer' to young people's disengagement, though it may support the development of the skills and literacies required for engagement. Thus we conclude that the broad decline in youth participation might be better redressed through offline initiatives designed to strengthen the opportunities structures of young people's lives and the 'communities of practice' (Wenger, 1998) available to them. This may prove more effective than building websites which, though they will engage a few, will struggle to reach the majority or, more important, to connect that majority to those with power over their lives in a manner that young people themselves judge effective and consequential.

Notes

1 These figures suggest a tendency to overclaim, since voting figures for the 2005 UK general election show that only 37 per cent of 18- to 24-year-olds and 48 per cent of 25- to 34-year-olds voted, compared with 71 per cent of those aged 55–64, and 75 per cent of those 65+ (Electoral Commission, 2005). There was a significant decline in young people voting in the 2001 general election (Hansard, 2001), and their interest in the political process is low (Haste, 2005; MORI, 2004). The issue of disconnection is complex, for there is some evidence of civic activism among the young alongside, or even in response to, their disenchantment from the formal political system (Bennett, 1998; MORI, 2004; Morris *et al.*, 2003).

2 Robert Putnam is perhaps the best known among those directly blaming rising public apathy and disengagement on the privatising effect of television on everyday life, with Robert Kraut having originally made a similar case for the Internet, though, as more people have gone online, altering the profile of users and uses, he has since revised this view (Kraut *et al.*, 2002).

3 Homes with children are fast acquiring multiple computers plus broadband access to the Internet. The UKCGO survey found that, in 2004, 36 per cent of 9- to 19-year-olds in the UK have more than one computer at home, and 24 per cent live in a household with broadband access. Furthermore, access platforms are diversifying: 87 per cent have a computer at home (71 per cent with Internet access), 62 per cent have digital television (17 per cent with Internet access), 82 per cent have a games console (8 per cent with Internet access) and 81 per cent have their own mobile phone (38 per cent with Internet access) (Livingstone and Bober, 2005).

4 As the latest Pew figures show (2005), this begins to rival time spent on any other medium, though not displacing time spent on social relations. For, increasingly, young people conduct their social relations through a multimedia mix of online, offline, face-to-face and mobile phone communication that reconfigures, but does not simply reduce, the degree to which young people are in touch with others.

5 In Couldry *et al.* (2007a), we define 'public connection' as 'the sense that, as citizens, we share an orientation to a public world where matters of shared concern are, or at least should be, addressed'.

6 The transition to adulthood is both a psychological and a sociological matter (Coleman, 1993), raising issues of developing identity, agency and commitment as well as those of enabling structures and institutional responses to young people's participation (Livingstone, 2002).

7 Indeed, since many rely on the main news 'brands' online, the content thus obtained may not differ greatly from broadcast news (Tewksbury, 2003).

8 Bentivegna (2002) summarises the view of many that the Internet is 'democratic' in that, while each of its features (interactivity, facilitated horizontal communication, disintermediation, reduced entry costs for small groups/individuals, and increased speed and flexibility of transmission and circulation) are not intrinsically new, when combined they enable the Internet to introduce a qualitative shift in the potential for democratic communication.

9 Response to the question, 'You are generally interested in what's going on in politics', measured – as are all the scales in this table – on a scale where 1 = strongly disagree and 5 = strongly agree.

10 Political Trust is a scale (Cronbach's alpha = 0.76) constructed following a factor analysis of three questions: 'You trust politicians to tell the truth', 'You trust politicians to deal with the things that matter' and 'You trust the government to do what is right.'

11 The political efficacy variable is the mean of responses to two questions: 'You feel that you can influence decisions in your area' and 'You can affect things by getting involved in issues you care about' which are significantly correlated (beta = 0.33, $p < 0.01$).

12 Three Social Capital questions were combined, following a factor analysis (Cronbach's alpha = 0.61): 'You play an active role in one or more voluntary, local or political organisations', 'Being involved in your local neighbourhood is important to you' and 'You are involved in voluntary work.'

13 Scale constructed from responses to the questions: 'People at work would expect you to know what's going on in the world' and, 'Your friends would expect you to know what's going on in the world', which are significantly correlated (beta = 0.51, $p < 0.01$).

14 The media trust scale (Cronbach's alpha = 0.65) is the mean of four variables (1 = strongly disagree to 5 = strongly agree): 'You trust the television to report the news fairly', 'You trust the press to report the news fairly', 'You trust the Internet to report the news fairly', 'You trust the media to cover the things that matter to you.'

15 The media literacy variable is the mean of responses to two questions: 'Different sources of news tend to give different accounts of what's going on' and 'You generally compare the news on different channels, newspapers or websites' which are significantly correlated (beta = 0.19, $p < 0.01$).

16 In a multiple regression aiming to predict interest in politics, neither overall amount of Internet use nor using the Internet as a news source added to the equation. What did predict political interest, with an R-squared of 29 per cent, were news engagement (beta = 0.33), class (–0.10: higher SES predicts higher interest), interest in celebrity (negatively, beta = –0.13), talking about issues (0.10), time spent reading a newspaper (0.08), listening to radio news (0.08), social capital (0.08) and media efficacy (0.08) – see Couldry *et al.*, (in press-a).

17 Anisah was initially visited as part of the 'Families and the Internet' project (Livingstone and Bovill, 2001) and then revisited as part of the 'UK Children Go Online' project (Livingstone and Bober, 2005). Mary was visited on both occasions as part of the Public Connection project (Couldry *et al.*, 2006).

3 New media and new voters

Young people, the Internet and the 2005 UK election campaign

Gustavo S. Mesch and
Stephen Coleman

Recent years have witnessed an increasing public and academic concern in western societies about the political participation of young adults. There is growing evidence that the turnout rate for 18- to 24-year-olds is decreasing from election to election. A Canadian study has shown that only about one quarter of the eligible 18- to 24-year-olds voted in the 2000 election (Pammett and LeDuc, 2003). In the UK a study by the Electoral Commission concluded that young people were half as likely to vote as older age groups and estimated that turnout among young people was lower in the 2005 general election than in 2001. According to a MORI study, it was 37 per cent compared to 39 per cent four years earlier (The Electoral Commission, 2005).

It is no surprise, therefore, that social scientists are interested in understanding the meaning of this continuous disengagement of young people from politics and the democratic system (O'Toole *et al.*, 2003; Kimberlee, 2002; Livingstone and Helsper, 2005). A central reason for these concerns is that this development calls into question the legitimacy of the political system itself, as a democratically elected government is supposed to be representative of the electorate. Any political system in which a large section of the population is either unwilling or unable to participate is not satisfactorily representative. Similarly, an elected government's mandate is diminished if their position is supported by an increasingly smaller section of the voting population. Thus, there is a danger of a downward cycle emerging, whereby candidates and parties focus their attention on groups who are likely to vote, to the neglect of those groups with lower turnouts. This, in turn, can lead to further alienation and decreased participation, as excluded groups feel that their legitimate concerns and interests are not represented. In addition, young people have differing political interests from older sections of the population, so lack of participation might prevent their generational interests and values from being represented (Henn *et al.*, 2002). If non-participation based on alienation and apathy is not addressed at an early age, some young people may get into a lifelong habit of not voting.

The rapid expansion in the use of ICTs has changed the way in which young people access information and communicate with peers, friends and family. Information sources are diversified, providing individuals with opportunities to access at any time, in real time, a larger variety of information sources and communication channels other than those provided by newspapers and television channels. The Internet also increases communication flexibility and permits users to exchange large amounts of information, regardless of geographic distance, facilitating communication with like-minded individuals and groups. Studies on the effect of the Internet on political participation are divided in their conclusions. Some have shown that the Internet is a well-suited technology for politically mobilising groups that were previously reluctant to participate in politics (Krueger, 2002). Others suggest that the Internet has done little to expand political participation to new individuals, but merely reinforces long-established patterns of participatory inequality (Livingstone and Helsper, 2005; Murdock and Golding, 1989)

The aim of the current study is to investigate differences in uses of the Internet for political purposes by young people in the 2005 UK general election. Previous studies have been limited in two aspects. First, they have investigated Internet use for politically-related activities between election periods. Thus, there is a lack of knowledge of how Internet users take advantage of ICTs for accessing politically relevant information and communicating with others in the context of voting in a public election. Our study is unique in that it investigates how individuals have used the Internet during a national election campaign. Second, the reinforcement thesis, which argues that the Internet merely reflects or amplifies, existing inequalities in the political system, was tested comparing individuals who had access with those who did not. Reinforcement effects in such studies may merely reflect inequalities of access which are then presented as inequalities of participation. Investigating existing users' use of the Internet during an election campaign provides us with an opportunity to uncover differences within the existing online population. Finally, we join the debate on youth political disengagement by exploring whether this group differs from the older population in their politically related use of the Internet during a political campaign.

The decrease in youth political participation

Current discourse on the decline of youth engagement in politics has mostly relied on two indicators: voting behaviour and party membership. These have been taken as key indicators of full participation in political deliberation and collective action (Kimberlee, 2002; Dahlgren, 2005). Yet, in recent years it has been recognised by academics and others that the decline in the involvement of youth in formal politics does not necessarily mean disinterest with politics per se (Henn *et al.*, 2002; Livingstone and

Helsper, 2005). Instead, some scholars have argued that young people are concerned with issues that are essentially political, but that these concerns and forms of expression are beyond the conventional indicators of political participation, such as voting turnout. Studies show that youth are the most likely to go online in search of information about politics (Gidengil *et al.*, 2003). Youth are involved in political issues that are not always closely tied to election campaigns, such as civil rights and environmental concerns (Mulgan and Wilkinson, 1997; Kimberlee, 1998).

There seems to be an agreement that the decline in voting and formal political participation by the young generation reflects contextual changes associated with the information society. Castells (2000), when developing the concept of a network society, noted that the structural changes that are characteristic of the information age are also reflected in institutional arrangements in the sphere of relations of production and consumption and in power relationships. He argues that historically social power was embedded in organisations and institutions organised around a hierarchy of centres, but that in the information age social organisation has shifted towards networks that are characterised by a more dispersed and shifting structure of power. This shift has a fundamental effect on politics: in western countries media have become the space of politics. In the information age, people access information required to consolidate their political opinion from electronic media that provide very simple, image-based political messages. Political discourse and competition is less focused on ideologies and political parties and more and more on individual leaders. Thus, there is a trend toward a personalisation of politics, with a focus on both political leaders and messages transmitted in the media. At the same time, individuals move from public spheres of debate and collective political gatherings as sources of information, to more personalised forms of access to political information and deliberation. Thus, it seems that in the information age there is a shift away from participatory politics; political parties seem less equipped to embrace, foster and nurture new, young activists, creating a feeling that much of mainstream political debate is now conditioned by the work of image makers and strategic advisers whose main task is to build political figures able to communicate simple messages through electronic media. In this new political situation, ICTs perform a specific role in facilitating personalised access to politically related information, political communication and collective mobilization.

ICTs and youth political participation

As the percentage of individuals with access to ICTs has increased, with higher rates of access and competence among the young generation, there are expectations that youth will use the Internet more effectively to access political information and as a public sphere for political debate and political activism (Gidengil *et al.*, 2003).

In exploring the potential effects of Internet use on political participation, it is important to highlight two different accounts and explanations (Norris, 2004). The mobilisation thesis emphasises the many interactive features of the Internet and claims that access to the Internet facilitates and encourages new forms of political activism. The strongest claims of mobilisation theorists are that net activism represents a distinctive type of political participation, which differs in many ways from conventional activities, like working for political parties, organising grass-roots social movements or lobbying elected officials. The Internet is conceived as a technology that reduces barriers to information access and dissemination and widens opportunities for political debate, encouraging group interaction. These technological affordances have led many organisations to develop websites, online forums and chat spaces which aim to encourage young people to make use of a wide range of opportunities online. The expectation is that among Internet users, youth will be more active in searching for information, interacting politically and using communication tools to influence others' political behaviour.

In contrast, the reinforcement thesis asserts that Internet use is strengthening rather than radically transforming existing patterns of political participation. From this more sceptical perspective, the Internet will serve to reinforce and perhaps even widen participation gaps between social groups (Livingstone and Helsper, 2005). Furthermore, it seems that Internet activists are a self-selecting group, so that the Internet does not change people, but simply allows them to perform traditional activities in a different way. Thus, while there have been some interesting changes in the way democracy works, the overall impact of ICTs is modest, and not yet deemed to be a transformative factor. As Margolis and Resnick (2000) concluded, there is an extensive political life on the net, but it is mostly an extension of that life off the net. While the major political actors may engage in online campaigning, lobbying, policy advocacy and organising, this perspective emphasises that there does not seem to be any major political change in sight and that the Internet has not made much of a difference in the political landscape; it has not helped to mobilise more citizens to participate, nor has it altered the ways that politics is conducted. Following this thesis, it would seem reasonable to expect that age differences in political participation observed offline will be reflected and reproduced online. Thus, youth will be less likely to search for political information, less prone to communicate with significant others and less likely to try to influence others in their political behaviour.

It is very likely that we are now in a transitional era of the information age in which the certitudes of the past with regard to how democracy works have become destabilised. Democracy is seen to be, precariously, at a new historical juncture (Castells, 2000). There has been a massive growth in online advocacy and issue politics, sometimes promoted by large and powerful interest groups, sometimes taking the form of grass-roots social movements, which represent characteristics of emerging, networked politics. It is often commented that the ostensible political disengagement from the established political system by many citizens may not necessary signal a disinterest in politics per se. Rather, many citizens have refocused their political attention outside the parliamentary system or they are in the process of redefining just what constitutes the political, often within the context of sociocultural movements. In the arena of new politics, the Internet becomes not only relevant, but central, giving rise to hopes relating to the capacity for horizontal communication and civic interaction within a new kind of public sphere (Dahlgren, 2005).

Following the literature review, the research question of the current study is whether online political participation reinforces or reflects the observed pattern of decline in political participation of the youth. The current study analyses data from a large sample of Internet users, according to age categories, and investigates the extent to which there is a generational gap in the use of ICTs for information access, interpersonal political communication and political activism.

Data collection

As the central question of the study was to investigate age differences among Internet users during the 2005 UK general election campaign, data was collected by an online polling company, YouGov, which was commissioned to conduct a survey of British citizens aged over 18 with access to the Internet. The polling company has built up a panel of more than 40,000 electors in the UK, recruited from a variety of non-political websites. Although the panel is not representative of the British public, as online users are not representative of the entire population, it includes enough subjects in each demographic group to provide opportunities for an in-depth analysis. Furthermore, previous studies have described differences among Internet users and non-users, concluding that Internet users seem to be more politically engaged than non-users. The use of an online-only survey controls for access differences and permits us to elaborate more on the differences within the existing online population.

Potential survey respondents completed a detailed questionnaire when registering with the company, based on which a representative sample of Internet-using electors was selected. Selected panel members were sent an email inviting them to complete a survey by clicking on an Internet link. Each panel member had a unique password to ensure that only the chosen respondents completed the survey. The response rates for our survey were 40 per cent on the first day and 60 per cent after 72 hours. Overall, 3,951 individuals completed the survey. The average age of respondents was 45 (ranging from 18 to 76) and 54 per cent were males.

The survey was conducted online in the week after the election. We are aware that Internet collection data have been received with suspicion, ranging from concerns of bias to upper-middle-class respondents to non-serious responses as an effect of respondent anonymity (Gosling *et al.*, 2004). Previous studies have shown that participants in online panel surveys are more politically interested and have firmer views on politics than those who have Internet access, but are not recruited to panels (Baker *et al.*, 2003; Gibson and McAllister, 2002). A comprehensive review comparing Internet-collected data with traditional methods concludes that data collected from Internet methods are not as flawed as is commonly believed and traditional methods are not inherently superior to Internet methods (Gosling *et al.*, 2004) While we do not think that use of the Internet should replace traditional methods in all instances, given our research goals, data collected via the Internet is appropriate for the current study.

Measures

As one of the central goals of the study was to investigate age differences in politically related Internet use, a variable measuring young and older participants was created. Youth was defined as individuals aged 18–25 and 'older people' were defined as participants in the age category 26–75. We adopted this definition as the 18–25 age group is the least likely to vote or participate in formal politics, according to most studies.

The survey included items measuring the extent of respondents' political interest. Respondents were asked to indicate the extent of their interest in the election and the extent to which they felt they had a duty to find information about the election. All the items were measured on a scale from 1 to 5, with higher scores representing higher interest. In addition, respondents were asked whether they had cast a vote in the 2005 election. Three types of Internet use during the election were studied. *Information* access was measured by questions asking about the extent to which the Internet was used to keep up with the news; to access campaign information on demand; and to access more reliable information than that supplied by broadcasters or the press. Internet use for *communication* was measured by questions asking about the extent to which respondents used the Internet to connect with others; and to send or receive emails related to the election campaign. Internet use for *political influence* was measured by questions about the extent to which respondents used the Internet to influence others, for example, by trying to persuade them to vote for the party they support.

In the multivariate analysis, two well-known variables that might influence political behavior, namely gender and socioeconomic status, were included as control variables.

Findings

Table 3.1 presents differences in the average responses to questions about voting behaviour and political interest. Youth and older people do

Table 3.1 T-test for differences in the means of items on electoral interest and voting behaviour

Variables	Older	Younger
Electoral interest and voting		
I was very interested in the elections	2.456	2.408
As a citizen I have a duty to find out about the election	7.383	6.853**
The Internet allowelïd me to influence other people	1.951	2.251**
I tried to influence other people to vote for the party I support	3.653	4.350**
I cast my vote in the 2005 election	0.867	0.673**

**$p < 0.01$

not differ statistically in their level of interest expressed in the election. In general, it should be noted that both groups were similar in expressing a relatively low interest in the election. The range of responses to the item was from 0 to 5 and the average in both cases is 2.4, indicating just an average interest.

However, there are clear generational differences in the perception of citizenship duties. The older generation is more likely to be committed to the electoral process, as such. This can be grasped from their responses to questions about the duty of citizens to seek election information and then vote. In response to both of these questions, older respondents express a stronger commitment to a civic duty of finding out about the election and a higher proportion of them have cast their vote. Only 67.3 per cent of the youth group voted in the election while 86.7 per cent of the older group of Internet users reported doing so.

At the same time, it should be noted that the results do not appear to be clear cut. While the older generation appears to express a more personal sense of voting duties, the younger generation appears to be more committed to active political communication and discussion. Members of the younger generation report higher average values in response to the question asking about the extent to which they tried to influence the voting behaviour of other individuals. In addition, members of the younger generation reported a higher average value in the extent that they tried to influence other people to vote for the party they support. Thus, while the younger generation seems to be less committed to casting votes, the results show that this is not a result of political indifference or disengagement. The young generation seems to be highly active in discussing political issues and even in trying to mobilise support for their chosen parties. This result supports critiques of measuring political engagement by using measures of voting behaviour alone. The results call for more research to explore why political engagement, as expressed in using the ICTs to air views and to convince others to vote for a particular party, is not translated into greater interest in the election campaign and in vote casting. One possible explanation is a gap between the perception of the consequences of being involved in public debate and the efficacy of the act of voting. In particular, when the results of the election seem to be known beforehand and personal participation in the voting process seems unlikely to make a real difference in the results, this can present a barrier to voting behaviour.

All political participation is based on access to information which provides the basis for the crystallisation of political preferences and opinion. We now turn to the analysis of generational differences in Internet use for the purpose of accessing information.

Table 3.2 presents the differences in the mean use of the Internet for information gathering purposes. The results show clear generational differences. It is clear that the young generation perceived the Internet as an important media channel for accessing information relevant to the election campaign. The first two items show that young people took advantage of the Internet to keep up with election news and to access information on demand. In fact, the average is relatively high and shows that youth were seeking information in a more temporally flexible fashion than the older generation. Furthermore, it seems that youth place less trust in the content provided by newspapers and television and use the Internet to access a more diversified range of information. In other words, the potential for more diverse, and possibly inclusive, views is higher online, and youth turn more frequently to this medium than the older generation.

Table 3.2 T-test for age differences in the use of the Internet for information gathering on the election

	Older	*Younger*
Information use of the Internet		
To keep up with the news about the election	2.904	3.305**
To access information whenever I need it	3.161	3.473**
To access a more reliable range of information than on the tv or the press	2.721	2.949**
To connect with others on campaigning issues	1.951	2.251**

**p < 0.01

Political involvement is a social process in which individuals meet each other to exchange views and information. In recent years this public sphere has weakened and declined, as political parties are less likely to organise mass meetings and there are fewer opportunities for face-to-face political interaction. Young respondents were more likely than older respondents to take advantage of the interactivity of the Internet to connect with others online and discuss political issues. It appears that for young Internet users, during the election campaigns, the Internet represents a type of new public sphere.

In the next battery of questions we were interested in respondents' specific online activities during the election campaign. The findings presented in Table 3.3 represent the proportion of respondents that reported doing specific activities during the election. A minority of Internet users did visit party websites, with marked generational differences: 40 per cent of the youth and 27 per cent of older respondents visited at least one party website. As found previously, the most frequent use of the Internet during the election campaign was for the purpose of finding information. This is corroborated in Table 3.3 where it can be seen that 60 per cent of the youth and 54 per cent of the older generation visited a news website. Of all the news websites, the BBC website was by far the one with the highest proportion of visitors that are Internet users, with 70 per cent of the youth and 56 per cent of older respondents reporting doing so.

A key normative function of political communication between citizens is that it allows them to exchange views and create political identities through discussion. The extent to which citizens go online for such purposes remains very limited. Only 14 per cent of young people and 13 per cent of older people report sending or receiving politically related emails. Paradoxically, although email is the most common form of Internet use, in relation to the election most Internet users went online to gather information and keep updated with the news rather than to exchange emails.

Table 3.3 T-test comparing proportion of respondents using the Internet for different political activities

Please indicate which of the following you have done during the election	*Young adults*	*Adults*
Visited a party website	0.401	0.275*
Visited a candidate website	0.176	0.159
Visited a news website	0.604	0.546*
Sent an email on the election	0.146	0.135
Received an email on the election	0.143	0.134

*$p < 0.01$

In order to gain a better understanding of the ways in which the different generations used the Internet during the 2005 election campaign, we were interested to find out how respondents themselves perceived ICTs as a politically enabling technology. Table 3.4 presents the results of questions asking about the extent to which the Internet enabled respondents to do different things, according to age.

The most conspicuous result here is the existence of consistent age differences in the perception of the utility of the Internet for different activities. The first three items refer to the extent to which Internet use enabled respondents to be more involved in the electoral campaign. A higher proportion of young than older respondents reported that the Internet enabled them to find information about the candidates and to gain a better understanding of the election issues. Probably the most frequent use reported by all respondents was the search for information on demand

Table 3.4 Percentage of respondents reporting extent that the Internet was used for certain activities

As a voter the Internet enabled me . . .		*Many times*	*A few times*	*Not many times*	*Not at all*	
To find out what candidates stand for	Elderly	6.6	31.4	30.6	31.4	100.0
	Young	16.7	35.4	26.6	21.4	100.0
To get as much information as possible about the candidates	Elderly	7.5	28.2	32.1	32.2	100.0
	Young	14.2	32.9	30.8	22.1	100.0
To get a better understanding of the central issues	Elderly	16.8	42.8	22.4	18.0	100.0
	Young	30.8	42.5	17.5	9.2	100.0
To be informed on the latest news on the campaign	Elderly	34.5	39.2	16.4	9.9	100.0
	Young	43.8	37.5	14.2	4.6	100.0
To get information faster than on the TV and newspapers	Elderly	36.7	36.6	14.4	12.2	100.0
	Young	42.9	34.6	12.9	9.6	100.0
To get multiple sources or viewpoints	Elderly	19.0	32.3	25.8	23.0	100.0
	Young	21.7	36.7	22.9	18.8	100.0
To help campaign for my candidate	Elderly	3.6	4.8	10.0	81.6	100.0
	Young	7.1	11.3	15.0	66.7	100.0
To donate to my party	Elderly	1.3	2.2	6.6	89.9	100.0
	Young	3.3	6.3	10.0	80.4	100.0
To communicate with like minded people about the election	Elderly	4.8	9.8	16.7	68.7	100.0
	Young	7.1	14.6	18.8	59.6	100.0
To communicate with friends and discuss politics	Elderly	6.0	10.6	16.4	67.0	100.0
	Young	10.0	20.4	15.8	53.3	100.0
To communicate with family and discuss politics	Elderly	4.0	7.9	15.3	72.7	100.0
	Young	7.9	15.8	12.1	64.2	100.0

at any time. Here again, young people placed greater emphasis upon this than older respondents.

A small group of respondents reported using the Internet for more active political purposes. The Internet enabled this small group to campaign for their chosen party or candidate, and communicate with like-minded, friends and family with a view to influencing them politically. But less than 10 per cent of respondents reported doing this frequently, with a higher percentage of young than older respondents reporting doing so.

In sum, it would seem from an initial scrutiny of the survey data that younger Internet users went online more frequently during the election campaign to access information at any time and influence political outcomes. Yet these descriptive results might be the result of other processes. For example, it might be that there are socioeconomic and gender differences that can account for this generational gap. In order to control for the possibility of intervening variables, we conducted a multivariate analysis which controlled for other demographic and attitudinal variables. The results are presented in Table 3.5.

The results of the multivariate analysis show that in both cases – as an information search and as a tool for political influence – the Internet is more likely to be used by the younger generation. Yet the results are not supportive of the mobilisation approach. Females and low-income individuals are less likely to use the Internet to search for political information

Table 3.5 OLS regression analysis of the characteristics of Internet users for communication and political influence purposes

Variable name	Searching for Internet information		Using the Internet to influence others voting	
Age (1 = young)	0.851 (0.175)	0.107**	0.314 (0.108)	0.064**
Gender (1 = male)	0.439 (0.106)	0.090**	0.146 (0.065)	0.049*
Socioeconomic status	−0.262 (0.106)	−0.054*	0.102 (0.065)	0.034
Interest in the election	0.553 (0.117)	0.106**	0.080 (0.072)	0.025
Perception of citizen duty	0.117 (0.024)	0.108**	0.026 (0.015)	0.039
Perception that online discussions are important	0.254 (0.025)	0.234**	0.161 (0.015)	0.241**
Constant	5.275** (0.362)		2.294** (0.223)	
Adj. R square	0.103		0.106	

or to use the Internet to influence others politically, regardless of age. This finding clearly demonstrates that even among a population of Internet users, gender and class differences that are well documented in the literature on offline political participation are reproduced. Furthermore, controlling for gender, socioeconomic status and age, political awareness, in terms of perceiving participation in elections a civic duty and perceiving online discussion as an important source for learning about politics, is positively related to Internet use, both for accessing information and influencing others.

Discussion

The results of the current study shed light on patterns of Internet use during an election campaign. One salient finding is the existence of a digital generation gap in the extent and frequency of use of new media. Young people rely on the Internet more than older people to access politically related information. Even when controlling for gender, socioeconomic status and attitudes that express interest in politics, young Internet users are more likely than older users to visit news-related websites and seek information about the parties and candidates. This finding suggests the value of Internet-based strategies by parties, candidates and media directed at including younger people, who are currently less likely to engage in election activities, while at the same time maintaining traditional mass-communication for the older generations who are less likely to be reached online. Yet our findings suggest that, even though young people are more likely to go online in order to interact with and influence others, such interactivity, which involves sending and receiving politically related emails, is under-utilised and generation differences are fairly small.

The findings provide partial support for the mobilisation hypothesis. Recent studies in western countries have consistently described a continuous decrease in electoral participation in elections and particularly low levels of political participation among younger people. Our findings, restricted to Internet users in the UK during the 2005 election, do not show that this political disengagement attributed to youth is reflected in their use of the Internet. For both accessing information, communicating about the election to others and attempting to influence the voting behaviour of others, young people seem to be more politically engaged when they are Internet users. Rather than reinforcing offline generational differences, it seems that the Internet is a medium which stimulates greater political engagement among young people.

Other findings in our analysis provide support for the reinforcement hypothesis suggesting that Internet use reflects traditional gaps between groups in political participation. Socioeconomic and gender differences observed in offline participation seem to be reflected and reproduced in the low level of election-related Internet use by females and less-educated individuals.

One finding appears to be paradoxical and requires further investigation. The population of the current study appears to be a more politically involved group. This can be inferred from the percentage of individuals that claim that they had cast their vote in the election. The percentage is higher than for the total population of the UK but at the same time, youth are less likely to have voted than the elderly. The paradox is that while youth use the Internet more than the elderly for accessing information, communication and influence the percentage that voted is lower than the percentage among the elderly. The finding appears to support the critique that measuring political interest only by voting behaviour is not warranted. But the paradox remains that despite more frequent access to campaign information and communication, this political interest was not translated in voting behaviour. One explanation might be structural, as in the last UK election it was clear from the beginning that the leading party would win and the prime minister re-elected. In that sense it was a situation in which the results were known beforehand. Under these conditions the motivation for voting decreases. But this explanation does not account for why this effect is much higher among the youth than among the elderly – a question that requires further investigation.

In the information age, political participation is moving away from involvement in institutionalised activities organised by political parties, to a more flexible political participation through individualised access to information and electronic social interaction. Compared to other age groups, the youth follow this process away from participatory politics, taking more advantage of ICT's that support their need for information, communication and influence at any time and from any place. The more individualistic nature of participation requires the adaptation of the political system. The political system needs to adapt by providing more individualised opportunities for social and political participation that are beyond strict partisan politics and strict face-to-face political gatherings.

At the same time, the results of the current study call for an evaluation of the low use of the Internet for political information and influence by women and less-educated individuals. Women and less-educated users seem to be less involved in accessing political information and less engaged in political communication. The risk that ICT might reinforce the political disengagement of these groups should be addressed in future studies with a goal of increasing our understanding of ways to reverse this trend and suggesting ways to reverse it.

4 Young voters and the web of politics

The promise and problems of youth-oriented political content on the web

Michael Xenos and W. Lance Bennett

Introduction

It is commonplace to refer to a crisis of youth participation in American electoral politics and in many other nations as well. Recent citizen cohorts are easily characterised as coming up short on a number of traditional civic engagement indicators, especially voting (Putnam 2000). This pattern echoes through societies in which young people increasingly sense that politics and political discourse do not address them. Although it is impossible to identify true turnout rates by age group in any given year, Levine and Lopez estimate that in the 2000 US elections only 37 per cent of Americans aged 18 to 25 cast ballots, compared to the national average of 51 per cent.[1] In the off-year elections of 2002 and 1998, only 17 per cent of young Americans voted – significantly lower than the national turnout rate.[2] This is troubling, though perhaps unsurprising, given that relatively few candidates seem to make appeals to young voters, and the political consultants who have become brokers in the relationships between citizens and representatives feel that young people are hard to reach and even harder to convince. Research on political participation suggests that one of the most important elements in taking part in politics is being asked to do so in some way (Schier, 2000; Verba *et al.*, 1995).

Many are tempted to see digital media in general and the expanding role of new media in electoral politics as convenient remedies to these problems. Sites like Rock the Vote and the increasing sophistication of candidates' use of online campaigning give the impression that the interactive nature of web communication provides a tailor-made pathway for today's wired young citizens to (re)enter the political world. Our investigations in this area, however, reveal a more complex picture of promise alongside substantial unrealised opportunity. On the one hand, as discussed in the following section, there are a variety of factors that point to digital media applications as important positive developments for youth engagement. In line with this, our data show that the growth of youth-oriented political content on the web has indeed been unmistakable. A substantial number of sites (youth-oriented and otherwise) have emerged to offer detailed issue information, as well as other useful tools that simplify processes like registering to vote, donating money to political causes, and contacting elected officials. At the same time, however, we also find a number of less encouraging signs. Candidates and other political actors, for example, appear far less interested in using the web as a way to bring in younger voters than one might suspect, given the distribution of Internet users by age group. In addition, beyond the campaign arena, the youth political web sphere aimed at attracting young people to politics appears to be maturing in network terms, but the pathways to political – particularly electoral – engagement from these networks are poorly developed.

Participation and the promise of digital media

In many ways, the temptation to view digital media as a 'technical fix' for declining rates of youth political engagement enjoys substantial support. Studies of the effects of Internet use at the individual behavioural level, for example, have produced encouraging findings. Such research has demonstrated the potential of Internet communication to generate interest in political campaigns, candidates and information, as well as to stimulate greater participation (Iyengar and Jackman, 2003; Stromer-Galley and Foot, 2002; Sundar *et al.*, 2003; Tolbert and McNeal, 2003). Moreover, available survey evidence suggests a younger generation that is both immersed in digital media and showing signs of a renewed interest in public life. In a report on the civic health of the nation, researchers affiliated with CIRCLE (Center for Information and Research on Civic Learning and Engagement) heralded the appearance of a distinct new generation of citizens, born after 1976 and dubbed the DotNets, with more positive attitudes about the role of government than their predecessors and a number of other distinctively encouraging characteristics (Keeter *et al.*, 2002).

Additionally, developments in the 2004 US election also appear consistent with this hopeful interpretation. That election witnessed a dramatic surge in youth participation and engagement with the political process alongside great strides in the use of digital media in politics. Younger Americans were surprisingly engaged in the presidential contest. In particular, during the 2004 campaigns, younger citizens showed a marked increase in reading news of the election, talking about it with others, and thinking about the election and how the outcome might affect them (Andolina and Jenkins, 2004). Indeed, an MTV/CIRCLE poll conducted at the height of the campaign found four-fifths of young voters were paying attention to the presidential contest ('The 2004 Presidential Campaign and Young Voters,' CIRCLE Fact Sheet 2004). Perhaps most significantly, younger voters also turned out to the polls in record numbers not seen since Bill Clinton was first elected in 1992. Although at the close of the election many commentators were quick to point out that the proportion of total votes cast in 2004 estimated to have come from younger voters showed no difference from prior years (around 17 per cent, the same as in 2000), subsequent research has revealed that the overall turnout was up, and that there were significant increases in the proportion of young citizens participating in the election. Estimates based on exit polls from the 2004 elections suggest that over half of the eligible population under 30 voted, and that approximately 42.3 per cent of 18- to 24-year-olds voted in 2004, up from 36.5 per cent in 2000 ('Youth Voting in the 2004 Election,' CIRCLE Fact Sheet 2004). Although accompanied, and somewhat obscured, by increases in turnout among all age groups, these numbers reflect the highest rates of youth turnout and political engagement in over a decade.

At the same time, the role of digital media in American electoral politics also expanded, perhaps most dramatically evidenced by Howard Dean's innovative uses of Internet campaigning in the Democratic primary, which presented an alternative to the traditional 'war room' campaign in the form of what has been termed the new 'networked campaign' model, combining elements of traditional campaign strategy with elements of flexibility and openness that have become the signatures of new media campaigns (Iozzi and Bennett, 2003). By the start of the general election, both major party candidates for president were fielding state of the art campaign websites that supplemented traditional candidate web fare, such as biographies and issue statements, with newer features like blogs and greater use of multimedia and other interactive techniques (Williams *et al.*, 2005). What is more, online political information also broke into the mainstream media audience in 2004. An estimated 75 million Americans, representing 37 per cent of the adult population and over half of American Internet users, went online to get information about the campaigns and engage in the political process; a substantial number, 20 million, were using the Internet to monitor campaign developments daily up to the close of the election (Rainie *et al.*, 2005).

As optimists would expect, younger Americans were at the forefront of online political information-seeking in 2004, perhaps taking sites like Rock the Vote as their starting points. Though older demographics have demonstrated higher rates of Internet use in recent years, Americans aged 18–29 have often remained near the top of usage statistics (Cole *et al.*, 2003) and have distinguished themselves as early adopters of interactive technologies like instant messaging and chat from the beginning stages of Internet growth (Madden, 2003). Indeed, studies estimate that more than 80 per cent of 18- to 29-year-olds use the Internet, as compared to estimates of between 58 and 64 per cent for Americans aged 50–65, and 22–34 per cent of those 65 or older (Fox, 2004; Cole *et al.*, 2003). Use of the web for political information seeking among young people follows a similar pattern, with 28 per cent of 18- to 29-year-olds estimated to have received most of their information about the 2004 election from the Internet – up from 22 per cent in 2000, and a higher proportion than for any other age-group (Pew Research Center, 2004).

It is difficult to assess what combination of factors produced these increases in turnout and interest in the election among younger voters. But it would surely be a mistake to point only to the rise of digital information sites and youth web networks. The 2004 US election was characterised by an intensive ground war of canvassing and personal contact, aimed at turning out young voters. One non-partisan youth mobilisation organisation characterised this effort as the 'largest non-partisan grassroots youth voter campaign in history' (New Voter Project, 2004). However, questions remain as to what young people encounter when they go online for political information, and what pathways may be more or less conducive to political engagement in elections and other kinds of politics.

Exploring youth oriented political content on the web

In this study we explore questions concerning the extent to which youth oriented political portals and other digitally mediated political communication hold the potential to help reinvigorate political engagement among tech-savvy American youth. Specifically, in this chapter we pursue three broad research questions. First, drawing on Foot and Schneider's concept of the 'web sphere' (2002), we ask, what is the nature of the youth engagement web sphere – that collection of sites aimed at attracting young people to politics in general, but not sponsored by particular parties or electoral candidates? To address this question we identify the key political issues and topics discussed on youth politics sites that are not specifically related to partisan electoral campaigns, as well as the interactive features used to attract and retain young visitors and to facilitate greater political engagement. Second, to what extent does the electoral web sphere (especially candidate and party websites) speak to the interests and sensibilities of younger Americans? To get at this question, we compare the issues and features found on samples of candidate campaign sites to those found on the youth sites, and also explore the extent to which sites in the electoral web sphere 'reach out' to younger voters, as compared to other kinds of voters. Finally, given that its networked hyperlink structure is one of the defining characteristics of web communication, what are the network characteristics of the youth political web sphere, and to what extent are there linkages or navigational paths between the youth political web sphere and the wider electoral web sphere? Here we explore the extent to which youth political web networks provide useful pathways for young people to follow in search of information, opportunities for political participation, and campaigns and organisations that match their political interests.

Overall, exploring these questions empirically reveals a mixed picture, including a number of patterns that raise questions about digital media as a simple fix for youth disengagement. Most troubling, we found a surprising absence of content and features directed at young people in the candidate websites, and our examination of the network properties of youth political sites as a group revealed a pattern of adaptation to the digital media environment that, while making important strides, appears to lag behind the efforts other political actors to capitalise on the network potentials of the Internet. To address the first two questions we conducted extensive content analyses of sites produced by youth oriented political organisations as well as traditional political actors (candidates and parties), archived during the 2002 and 2004 elections. Additionally, to shed light on the third question we created a series of network maps of the youth political web sphere that chart the emergence and development of this unique part of the web over time. Together, we believe these observations suggest that while digital media provide some promising inroads to electoral participation for a largely disengaged younger generation, a number of important elements of this terrain must still be negotiated if that potential is to be fully realised.

Data and methods

Our data on the youth engagement web sphere come from comprehensive content analyses we conducted on archival copies of political engagement sites aimed at young people, collected during the 2002 and 2004 US election cycles. The political campaign web data come from two sources. During the 2002 cycle, we conducted content analysis of nearly 200 candidate campaign websites, which we compare to data from a smaller sample of 2004 campaign websites gathered by other researchers (Foot *et al.*, 2005).

Site identification and sampling

In each of the two election cycles under study, a collection of youth political engagement web sites was generated using a combination of site identification techniques. First, in each cycle a series of Google searches were conducted using descriptors such as 'youth', 'political', 'politics', 'elections', 'citizenship' and 'civic'. The site URLs generated in this process were then used to create a 'seed list' that was fed into the Issue Crawler tool developed by Richard Rogers.[3] The Issue Crawler identifies networks of sites based on linkages to, from, and among an original list of sites on the basis of co-link analysis. A co-link is simply a page that is linked to or from at least two of the starting points for that iteration. If a site is added to the list as a result of the co-link analysis, it then becomes one of the starting points for the next iteration. By adjusting the network parameters inputted into the crawler at the beginning of a crawl (for example, varying the seed lists of sites, the depth to which the crawler scans each site for links, and the number of iterations for each crawl), we were able to identify what we believe to be reasonably complete renderings of youth engagement site networks for each of the two election cycles, leading us to the final lists of sites that comprise what we consider to be the youth political web spheres for 2002 and 2004, and the primary data pool for our content analyses of youth sites.

Through each of the iterations of crawling, the goal was to identify portal sites focusing generally on political issues (rather than narrowly on one issue, or one set of issues) and oriented toward the 18- to 24-year-old demographic group. We deleted from our analyses sites from interest organisations that did not display a clear youth engagement programme. We also added sites that were identified by other researchers working on youth engagement that did not emerge from the automated crawling process that generated our initial list. At every turn, we sought to create the most inclusive and exhaustive collection of websites providing political content directed primarily at younger citizens, guided by the principles of web sphere analysis outlined by Foot and Schneider (2002). Ultimately, the 2002 list included some 24 sites, and the 2004 sphere totalled 35 sites. After archiving the sites using an off-the-shelf web crawler program,[4] we were then able to conduct our content analyses on what we believe represent the full universes of youth political portals that operated in the US 2002 and 2004 election cycles.

Our primary set of political campaign candidate sites was drawn from the archival collection of all of the 2002 House, Senate and Gubernatorial candidate websites produced by Webarchivist.org and available at the Library of Congress under the Mapping the Internet Electronic Resources Virtual Archive (MINERVA) collection (http://www.loc.gov/minerva/), as well as through Webarchivist's public scholarship site, http://politicalweb.info. Although it is often the sites of presidential candidates that receive the most popular attention in discussions of online politics, our analysis proceeds from the assumption that the vast majority of campaigns in the United States are for these lesser offices. Indeed, at the height of the campaign season in 2002, over 1,600 individuals officially competed for House, Senate and Gubernatorial office, and nearly two-thirds of them fielded a functional, stand-alone campaign website (Foot *et al.*, 2002). Close to 1200 websites are included in the 2002 Election Web Archive.[5] Lacking the resources to conduct coding on the full universe of campaign sites from 2002, we opted for a random sample of just over 200 of the sites listed in the archive. Initial analyses of the make-up of the sample, focusing on the contexts within which each site was produced (for example, the partisanship of candidates, and their likelihood of success as gauged by campaign intensity), revealed no significant differences between our sample and the full universe of cases available in the archive. Ultimately, close to 30 sites were eliminated from coding due to exclusion of the actual site contents by the campaigns themselves,[6] problems with archival availability of the sites,[7] and in a few cases the mistaken inclusion in the archive of Web sites that were not official campaign sites.[8] In all, a total of 177 archival website impressions comprised our (hyper)text corpus for the candidate site content analysis.

Data on youth oriented content in the 2004 electoral web sphere were generously provided by Kirsten Foot and her collaborators, who allowed us to include an item on youth appeal in their more general analysis of web practices engaged in by political actors in the 2004 elections (Foot *et al.*, 2005, in press). In their analysis of the 2004 electoral web sphere, they used a similar process of focused sleuthing to identify a set of sites representing the web presence of a variety of different political actors. Based on the results of this site identification process, they then created a representative sample for coding purposes. Although smaller than our 2002 sample, their sample of the 2004 web sphere includes a total of 102 sites from four distinct producer types. Specifically, they coded candidate, party, labour organisation/NGO and press/portal sites. A fifth, 'other' category was also created for sites that did not fall cleanly into one of these four categories (for example, sites produced by individuals).

Coding

We coded the archival renderings of the youth engagement and election campaign websites as they appeared at the height of the 2002 campaign season, typically in late October or early November.[9] Graduate and undergraduate researchers conducted the coding using a web-based survey tool, which facilitated data transfer during the coding process.

Youth engagement sites

The coding scheme developed for the youth political sites probed for the presence or absence of 16 distinct political issues, and 15 specific features. The list of issues was developed on the basis of polling data identifying the political issues salient to voters during the time period for which we coded the websites. These 'most important problem' data included traditional national samples, as well as samples of voters aged 18–25 years. We also coded for a collection of website features to determine the extent to which various attractive features of the web (for example, blogs, links, personal logins and polls) were available in the respective web spheres. The list of features was developed on the basis of prior research on the 2002 candidate websites (Foot *et al.*, in press), as well as exploratory analyses of the youth sites themselves. Table 4.1 lists the specific issues and features included in the coding scheme. Overall, inter-coder percentage agreement for each of these items falls within the acceptable range, with the vast majority at or above 90 per cent.

Candidate sites

In order to address our second research question concerning the extent to which candidates and other political actors 'reach out' to younger voters,

Table 4.1 Issues and features coded in the youth engagement web spheres

Issues	Features
Education	Voter registration
Health Care	News/press releases
National security/terrorism	Photos
Taxes/government spending	Endorsements
Economy/Jobs	Email signup
Social security	Contact officials
Environment	Participation/mobilisation
Gun control	Multimedia content
Crime/violence	Send links
Abortion	Message board or blog
Campaign finance reform	Interactive polls
Minority rights/recognition	Contact media
Politics/government changes	Personal login
Censorship/free expression	Onsite information on elections
National debt	Links to information on elections
Gay rights	

our coding scheme for the 2002 candidate sites included items tapping the presence or absence of the same 16 issues and 15 features included in the youth site coding scheme.[10] This enabled us to compare the content and features of the two kinds of sites. Additionally, we also included a number of items probing for the presence of age-related appeals within both the issues content, and the features employed on the candidate sites. This enabled us to more fully assess the extent to which candidates reached out to youth sensibilities in 2002. To illustrate, for each distinct issue identified on a site, we asked coders to probe further for the presence of either *implicit* or *explicit* appeals to younger citizens. Implicit appeals were defined as the presence of photographs or other images that either featured individuals resembling members in the 18–25 year age group, or symbolised that group. For example, coders looked for photographs of young workers on pages related to the economy and college students on pages related to education. Explicit appeals were defined as direct, textual references to younger voters, where younger voters were clearly part of the intended audience. For example, under this system if a candidate posted to their site a block of text decrying the flight of young people from her rural district, this would not be coded as an explicit youth appeal on economic issues, whereas a different candidate page including calls for greater student loan funding to help younger constituents finance their educations would be coded as an explicit youth appeal on education. Ultimately, we found that implicit and explicit appeals to young people were so infrequent that we combined both into a single measure for presence of youth appeals in issue content, and inter-coder agreement was calculated on the basis of this combined measure. With respect to youth appeals in site feature content, we examined four distinct facets of the typical campaign website; we looked for explicit or implicit youth appeal or representation in:

- mobilisation/participation features (such as a campaign calendar featuring events held on college campuses);
- photo galleries;
- news items listed in a press release or newsroom section of a website;
- endorsements (for example, from the local College Republicans or College Democrats).

As a point of comparison, we also coded for the presence or absence of appeals to another age-based demographic, senior citizens, using similar procedures. Finally, we also coded for the presence of biographical sketches in the candidate websites. Inter-coder percentage agreement for each item in the candidate site coding displayed slightly more variation than those for the youth site coding, but were generally above 80 per cent.

As mentioned earlier, our 2004 electoral web sphere coding data come from an item included in Foot *et al.*'s (2005/forthcoming) analyses. This item was based on our original items on youth appeals in the 2002 candidate coding, but in keeping with our earlier findings combined references to implicit and explicit appeals. Other than this slight change, the wording and instructions for this item were taken from our original coding scheme. The result is a measure comparable to our collapsed 2002 variable, though somewhat less precise than our more elaborate coding of the 2002 candidate sites. It is important to note, however, that since this measure reflects a simple presence or absence of youth appeal on each site in general, it is therefore in some ways more sensitive toward the identification youth content.

Network properties of the youth political web sphere

Finally, to determine the emergence and chart any growth or development of networks in the youth political web sphere, we conducted a series of controlled crawls using the Issue Crawler at a number of different time points. These crawls provide a unique time-lapse picture of the youth political web sphere over time. For each of these crawls, we entered as a seed list the collection of sites identified as the youth engagement sphere for that election cycle, and instructed the crawler to go through two iterations of the co-link analysis described earlier, and to scan each site to a depth of two pages for links.

Findings: promise and problems

Our findings suggest a mixed picture about the promise of digital media for youth engagement. While consistent in important ways with a more optimistic view of the potential of digital media to provide promising pathways into electoral politics for younger citizens, our findings also highlight a number of problematic areas where the full potential of digital media appears to remain unrealised. The most promise is shown in the development of the youth political web sphere, beginning with the sheer volume of sites (from 22 sites identified in 2002, to 35 in 2004). There is also development in both issue content and features. Perhaps most importantly for realising the networking capacity of the web, our time-lapse pictures of sites in the youth engagement web sphere also show important signs of increasing sophistication. On the other hand, our analyses of candidate sites reveal a far less comforting picture. Although candidates often discuss issue topics that younger Americans are interested in, or at least appear on youth-oriented sites, there is little effort to address these in language or policy terms aimed at younger demographics (compared, for example, with clear attempts to target appeals to senior citizens). Even greater missed opportunities are revealed in the substantial gaps between the candidate and youth sphere sites in terms of the visual and interactive features offered. Moreover, we found that these differences also translated into a less than seamless integration of the two web spheres. We begin with the findings with the promising developments in the youth engagement sphere, and conclude with a look at the many missed opportunities in the election campaign sphere.

The youth engagement web sphere comes of age

As noted earlier, on the surface, the most observable pattern in the youth engagement web sphere during the time period under study was its marked increase in size, from 22 to 35 identifiable actors. Within this unique sphere of web content, we also find a vibrant array of information and features, as well as a number of encouraging signs of growth and development over time.

In terms of issues and informational content, we may begin by considering the simple case of offering a distinct menu of 'issues' information. For the 2002 youth engagement web sphere we detected pages devoted to information on a menu of political issues within only 8 of the 22 sites identified. By 2004, however, we found discussion of specific political issues on close to two-thirds of the 35 youth political websites identified in our 2004 analyses. Further comparisons of the sites from 2004 with those of 2002 also revealed greater levels of general information about the current elections, greater provision of information on voter registration, and greater levels of information about actual offline political events and opportunities for political participation. Indeed, by 2004 over half of the youth-oriented political websites examined contained information on the elections in some form, information on how to register to vote, and information about events and ways to get involved. Especially noteworthy across the two time points is the shift *away* from providing specific information about the elections through links to third-party sites, like the one produced by League of Women Voters, and *toward* the provision of election information on-site, in a context more directly targeted toward younger voters. These areas of growth, and the conversion of election information transmission from off-site links to on-site content, are graphically illustrated in Figure 4.1.

With respect to the features offered on youth oriented political websites, we also found a number of promising patterns. Though even in 2002 youth oriented political websites offered an impressive array of interactive and multimedia features, comparing analyses of features on these sites from both the 2002 and 2004 election cycles again reveals substantial gains during this time period. Although there were declines in two features from 2002 to 2004 – the use of interactive opinion polls and pages providing interactive forms that enable site visitors to contact elected officials – overall, we see a steady, and in some cases, marked increase in the presence of a

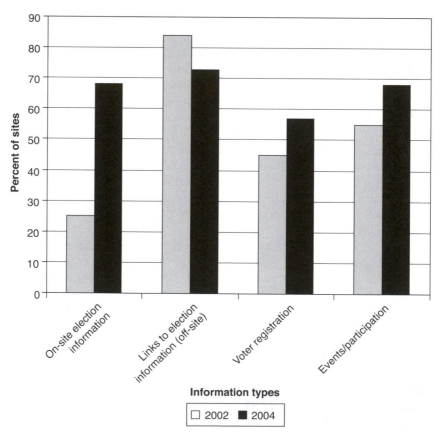

Figure 4.1 Political information provided on youth political websites, 2002–04
(*N* for 2002 sites: 22; *N* for 2004 sites: 35)

variety of web-exclusive communication techniques. The most common features found on youth sites in 2004 were sign-up forms for email updates, which alert visitors to new site content, news/press release pages, often highlighting events and issues of unique concern to younger voters, and photos, which often help young voters to identify with the producers of a given website. These three features were found on 81 per cent, 86 per cent, and 83 per cent of the youth political sites we coded in 2004, respectively. As in the broader world of Internet communication, there were also marked gains in the presence of message boards or blogs on youth political websites across the two time points, representing a 70 per cent increase over their prevalence in the 2002 cycle. The proportions of youth political websites containing these features in 2002 and 2004 are shown in Figure 4.2.

A final set of positive observations concerning the potential of digital media as a vehicle for youth political engagement comes from our investigation of the network structure of youth-oriented political websites as a group. The baseline for this comparison is starkly clear: our earliest attempts to map the network of youth political websites in 2002 produced such a sparsely networked collection of sites as to make mapping nearly impossible. However, on the basis of network maps generated over a period of ten months, including crawls before, during and after the 2004 election, we see that the collection of youth-oriented political websites experienced important advances in connectedness to the wider web of

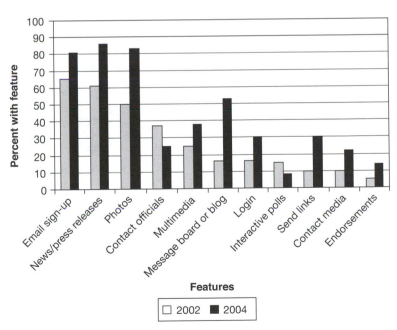

Figure 4.2 Features on youth political websites: 2002–04
(*N* for 2002 sites: 22; *N* for 2004 sites: 35)

political sites on the Internet. These advances are best illustrated through a comparison of the network map generated from our seed list of youth-oriented sites in July of 2004 (Figure 4.3), and the map generated using an identical seed list and set of parameters in November 2004, at the height of the campaign season (Figure 4.4).

In examining these maps and the more detailed matrix of linking patterns on which they are based, we see a number of important patterns in the linkages and navigational paths within the youth political web sphere, as well as connections to other sites featuring political content related to the elections. Comparing the July network to the November network, for example, we see a clear progression as the election drew closer: the network grows in size and complexity, eventually reaching a peak just before election day. In July, for example, five months preceding the election, we see a relatively sparsely populated map of network actors, with few of the sites comprising the youth engagement web sphere receiving links from other election network nodes, or connecting disparate regions of the network together. By November, the network topography has become highly compact, with youth oriented political websites occupying central positions within the broader network of election websites, and node locations on the map rendered much more densely with more links, indicating greater ease in terms of navigating from node to node. Although not shown, a

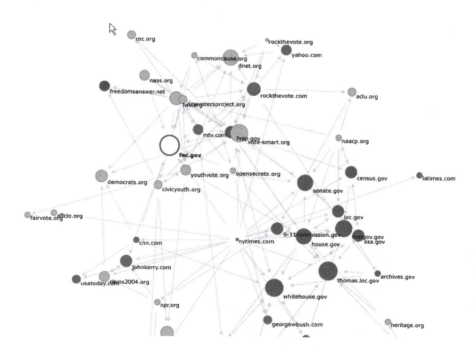

Figure 4.3 Network map of the youth engagement web sphere: July 2004

later map rendered in April 2005 depicts a moderate, though not total, relaxation of the network, exhibiting a level of activity and interlinking somewhere between the July and November maps.

In numerical terms, we may describe the network development between July and November by stating that in the July map, we see 50 sites represented, and a total of 173 links between those points, whereas in the November map we see 60 sites, and a total of 387 linkages. This represents more than twice the total number of links, and a substantial increase in the density of the network. On the whole then, we may say that although our earlier investigations of the network structure of the youth political web sphere in 2002 were somewhat uninspiring, the structure of pathways and linkages found during the 2004 election indicates a healthier pattern with respect to the Internet as a starting point for young citizens interested in the electoral process. This pattern may be an example of Bimber's notion of an increased agility and responsiveness among organisations within the post-bureaucratic political structure induced by new media (2003). In addition, the relatively self-organising emergence of a denser network by election day represents an interesting ecological dynamic in network structure (Monge, 2004). Focusing events such as elections may enable network nodes to connect in ways that may persist (to some degree) after the end of the activating events.

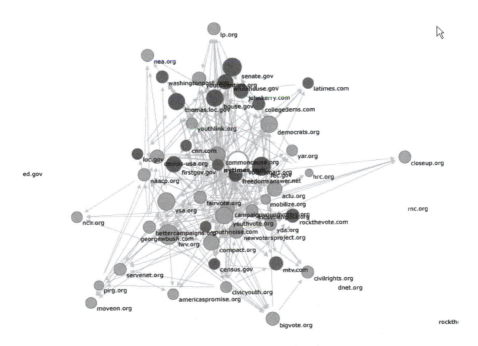

Figure 4.4 Network map of the youth engagement web sphere: November 2004

The electoral web sphere: missed connections

Turning our attention to the election websites, and the linkages between the youth and electoral web sphere, a number of findings and patterns complicate a conclusion that the web provides an easy pathway to voting and other forms of political engagement for young people. Specifically, we found a notable lack of appeals to young people and comparatively fewer features in the candidate sites. Moreover, the bridges between the youth engagement sphere and the electoral web sphere are still not well established.

Issues and features on candidate websites

As noted earlier, the broad topical focus of issues on the candidate sites analysed in 2002 was similar to that found in the youth sites. That is, young voters were likely to find discussion of the same kinds of issues (education, health care, national security/terrorism, taxes/spending and the economy) on candidate sites as they would on youth sites. There were a few exceptions to this pattern, for example issues like gun control (on roughly half of the youth sites but only 31 per cent of candidate sites) and gay/lesbian rights (also on roughly half of the youth sites but only found on 6.2 per cent of candidate sites), but the overall pattern is one of overlap. The critical divergence is in terms of the ways in which issues were discussed. Indeed, despite indications that young voters are the group most likely to go online to seek political information, particularly in contrast to senior citizens, we found that in 2002 the candidates rarely phrased or framed issues in ways that directly addressed young people.

First, we found a large number of issues on which candidates made no age-related appeals. On its own, this is a troubling finding, but one that may be less alarming if we assume that the absence of age-related appeals is a sign of age-neutrality rather than aversion to younger voters. However our data suggest that candidates often opt for an age-specific format in issue discourse. As a point of comparison we identified whether issue appeals on sites either directly or indirectly appealed to another age-based demographic, that of senior citizens, and found that candidates reached out to this group far more often. Of the 16 issues included in our study, half contained at least some appeal on the basis of age. The issue of greatest age specific appeal to young voters was the obvious issue of education, but even here, there were age specific appeals only in 23.3 per cent of the cases. Appeals to young people were all but non-existent on most of the other issues, and in terms of social security (which, considering the future of the programme, has great potential for youth appeals) and health care, senior appeals dwarfed youth appeals. In the case of social security, we found senior appeals over 70 per cent of the instances in which it was discussed, as compared to youth appeals, which were present in less than

20 per cent of the candidate pages on social security. For health care, the disparity runs from over 60 per cent of candidate issue pages featuring senior appeals, compared to less than 5 per cent featuring youth appeals.

Overall, we believe these findings speak clearly to the question of the extent to which candidates appear to be reaching out to younger voters in their online issue communications. The resounding answer is in the negative. Despite the fact that there appear to be no strategic costs associated with including youth appeals in online candidate statements on issues such as the environment, crime and violence, and economic growth and job creation, candidates in 2002 almost universally did not do so, reinforcing the common sentiment that younger voters who ignore politicians largely do so because politicians largely ignore them.

With respect to the features deployed on candidate websites in 2002, we found another, though less stark, point of disconnection. On the whole, candidates used very little of the interactive capacities of the web to reach voters in 2002. Candidates used interactive features much less often than producers of youth-oriented political websites. Indeed, our results are consistent with previous studies suggesting that candidates are much more likely to use the web as an efficient way of distributing basic information than they are to take advantage of its interactive and multimedia capabilities (Stromer-Galley, 2000; Foot *et al.*, 2002). The most common features found on candidate websites in 2002 were candidate biographies (87.6 per cent) and pages devoted to news items and press releases (57.1 per cent). Just over a third (35 per cent) offered an email newsletter. Multimedia content, message boards and interactive polls were found on fewer than 10 per cent of the candidate sites we coded.

Overall, we see that with the exception of endorsements, which are found much more frequently on candidate sites, the key points of divergence are precisely in the areas of interactive and multimedia features. Simply put, young voters visiting candidate sites in 2002 were unlikely to find the same kind of interactive environment they might have been accustomed to through exposure to political websites more directly targeted toward them. Though such features were not widespread among the youth political sites, they were certainly more common than in the mainstream political web. For example, youth sites featured online forums and other pages facilitating visitor communication with media (for example, writing letters to the editor) five times as often as candidate sites, and the youth sites featured interactive polls, multimedia content and message boards three times as often as candidate sites. In the features dimension, our conclusion is clear: candidates in 2002 used the interactive and multimedia features unique to the web environment much less frequently than the producers of youth political websites. Figure 4.5 provides an illustration of these key points of divergence.

As discussed earlier, we were not able to replicate the same extensive coding of candidate websites in 2004 as we had in 2002. However, drawing

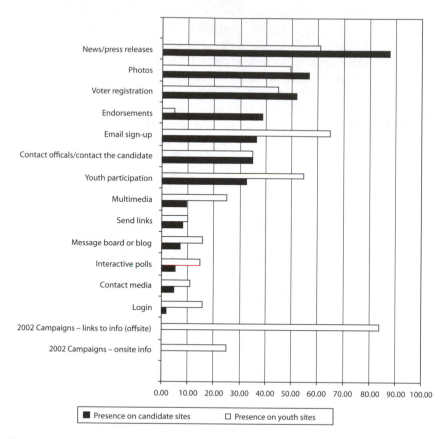

Figure 4.5 Features on youth vs. candidate political web sites (2002)

upon research and data from our colleagues, we were able to partially confirm whether the patterns just described transferred over into the 2004 political web sphere. These data, which come from a smaller number of sites but a greater variety of political actors, including political parties and interest groups advocating their issues in the election, suggest levels of issues discussion and features (such as email sign-up, multimedia content and voter registration) comparable to those found on candidate sites in 2002. With respect to youth appeals, these data from the broader electoral web sphere in 2004 show that the use of the web to reach out to younger voters by mainstream political actors continued to be quite sporadic, with only 8 per cent of all sites examined featuring some type of appeal to younger voters. Considering the slightly broader nature of our measures for youth appeal in 2004 as compared to those used in the 2002 analyses, this is hardly encouraging. Political party websites, however, did feature youth-targeted content at a non-trivial rate of 27 per cent, suggesting that mainstream political actors may be moving toward greater efforts to communicate through the web with its most avid and savvy users. However, in the other categories (labour/NGO, press and other) youth appeals were found at rates of 10 per cent or fewer. In the main then, these figures reinforce our findings from 2002 with respect to the puzzling paucity of appeals made by major actors in electoral politics to a substantial segment of those going online to seek political information.

Connecting the youth engagement sphere with the electoral web sphere

In addition to our more detailed quantitative coding, we also conducted a more informal investigation of the kinds of click-paths that would-be young voters may have followed from the sites of the youth political web sphere into the electoral web sphere. Though somewhat imprecise, these investigations led to some additional noteworthy observations on the potential of politics online to help reinvigorate levels of youth engagement in electoral politics. The overwhelming impression was one of pathways that were not as smooth as the basic co-link analyses from our network maps might suggest. For example, a young voter interested in social security reform may easily find information on that topic on a site like Rock the Vote, and even links to organisations working in this policy area. However, doubtless due to the non-partisan nature of these sites, very little interpretive information that might help match specific interests and geographic locations to particular candidates and campaigns is provided. Although we did find a shift, from 2002 to 2004, away from a simple link-menu strategy and toward providing more specific information on the youth sites themselves, in many cases, the experience following the personal discovery of a particular issue somewhere in the youth politics sphere is to dump the now motivated young citizen into a generic voter site like the League of Women Voters, where she must start from the beginning to learn about candidates' positions on the issue.

One promising exception was the strategy deployed by sites such as http://www.indyvoter.org, which used site features similar to those found on the dating and social networking websites popular among young Internet users that help connect younger citizens with others who share common interests and preferences. As configured during the 2004 elections, the indyvoter.org site featured a system through which 'joining' the website and obtaining a login also involved creating a user profile, complete with photos and biographical statements. Users could use the profiles to contact others, by interest or location, to share information and coordinate offline political actions. Perhaps most valuable, users were also encouraged to create their own personal or collective 'voter guides,' which were then made available to all other members. Though relatively unnoticed during the 2004 cycle, these innovations represent significant steps in terms of combining the features and functionality common to sites more frequently visited by younger citizens with political information and avenues to participation, but unfortunately were an exception that proved the rule with respect to greater use of the networking capabilities of the web to help young citizens connect with politics.

Conclusion

Based on this sketch of young people and politics in a digital age, one can find many positive developments contributing to the popular image of the Internet and associated technologies as a 'technical fix' to the problem of youth political (dis)engagement. But a variety of factors lead us to strongly caution against an interpretation that attributes the recent increase in youth electoral participation to greater and more sophisticated use of the Internet by political candidates, and a greater presence of the Internet in American politics more generally. These developments, though perhaps partly attributable to enhanced Internet communications and youth network infrastructure, were clearly the result of a complex array of institutional forces, many of which are entirely unrelated to online politics. One should not be surprised to note that youth turnout in 2004 was highest in the so-called 'battleground' or hotly-contested states, and likely fueled by some of the most intense canvassing and get-out-the-vote efforts in history (Lopez *et al.*, 2005). Indeed, based on the data presented here, we believe a sober account of the promise and potentialities of the web as a vehicle for youth political engagement must accept a set of mixed results. On one hand, the body of political information and resources targeted at younger voters online (what we refer to here as the youth political web sphere) has undergone important development in recent years. Based on analyses beginning in 2002, we believe the 2004 cycle was a critical moment in the development of online political infrastructure for American youth. But on the other, the candidate and campaign web sphere continues to be lacking in important content and features when compared to the youth political web sphere, and accessible pathways between the two spheres appear to remain short of their potential. If the Internet's true potential as a pathway to greater youth engagement in the political sphere is to be realised, it will be important to consider these issues and their evolution as interest and research in the areas of new media and politics continue.

Notes

1 As Levine and Lopez (2002) note, official Federal Election Commission data on ballots cast do not contain information on the age of voters. Thus, any estimate of turnout by age must be derived from survey data. Though such data are notorious for their inflation of voter turnout, the Census bureau data used by Levine and Lopez are collected within two weeks of each election and are thought to contain only a modest 10 per cent over reporting rate. Further, despite

the debates over appropriate measures of overall voter turnout (c.f. McDonald and Popkin), Levine and Lopez conclude that youth voting rates are low 'by any measure'.

2 2002 data from http://www.childtrendsdatabank.org/, 2000 data from Levine and Lopez (2002).

3 For information on the Issue Crawler, see http://www.govcom.org/crawler_ software.html

4 Specifically, we created an archival version of each site using *Teleport Pro*.

5 Though these numbers suggest a 75 per cent, rather than a 64 per cent rate of web presence, this discrepancy is due to the inclusion in the archive of websites produced by candidates who ran at one time during the 2002 season, but either dropped out of their races or were defeated in primary elections.

6 Candidates were, and are, able to remove their records from the archive collection in two ways; candidates may 'opt out' of the archive officially, or they may have included technical features on their sites (the robots.txt exclusion) that disable automated collection techniques, such as those used in the creation of the archive.

7 Though the technology has come a long way, web archiving continues to be a complex endeavour. As a result of the many variations in site design, layout, organisation and construction, as well as the occasional contingencies of the Internet itself, 100 per cent reliability remains on the horizon. We believe, however, that exclusion from our analysis on the basis of these factors exhibits no underlying systematic bias.

8 For example, a few candidates listed personal or professional web pages in their campaign documents – such as Martin Lindstedt, Republican Senatorial candidate for Missouri, whose archived site is not primarily dedicated to his Senatorial campaign.

9 Archival rendering allows one to view a site more or less exactly as it was rendered during the time period specified. When a site is collected into the archive the files associated with that site are captured and stored electronically. Each time this is done, an archival 'impression' is made of the site for that point in time. For example, most of the campaign sites used in the study were captured on a daily basis. Thus one can select a specific date from index pages at politicalweb.info or MINERVA at the Library of Congress and view the impression of the site, which reproduces it as it was seen by web surfers on that particular day.

10 For seven of the 15 features analysed we were able to obtain reliable estimates of their presence from prior research (Foot *et al.*, 2002) gathered on the basis of larger samples, thus these items were removed from our coding scheme.

5 Young activists, political horizons and the Internet

Adapting the net to one's purposes

Peter Dahlgren and Tobias Olsson

The Internet's significance for the life of democracy has been a recurrent theme within research, as well as in popular debates, for about a decade now (cf. Holmes, 1997; Poster, 1997; Hague and Loader, 1999; Hoff *et al.*, 2000; Margolis and Resnick, 2000; Meikle, 2002; Jenkins and Thornburn, 2003; Shane, 2004; Dahlgren and Olsson, 2007). Some of this literature emphasises traditional political parties (for example, Nixon and Johansson, 1999; Tops *et al.*, 2000; Anderson and Cornfield, 2003; Bimber and Davis, 2003; Gibson *et al.*, 2003). Other efforts have extra-parliamentarian settings as their focus (for example, Castells, 1997; Kahn and Kellner, 2004; McCaughey and Ayers, 2003; van de Donk *et al.*, 2004; de Jong *et al.*, 2005; Caemmerts and Carpentier, 2006). In addition, there have been efforts using statistical studies that have tried to present an overarching view of Internet's political significance through an analysis of the access to and the use of the Internet among various groups of users (cf. Wilhelm, 2000; Quan-Haase *et al.*, 2002).

These discussions – especially in the early days of Internet research – can be said to have a theoretical bias. Quite often they have started from an analysis of the new information and communication technology per se and then tried to estimate its political significance – they have, so to speak, read the new ICT's political significance off the technology itself. For instance, the Internet's network structure has been seen as a forerunner to a politics following network logic (for example, Barney, 2004; Hassan, 2004). Moreover, we suggest that a good deal of the relevant literature also suffers from a lack of a 'media perspective', not treating the net as part of a larger, integrated media environment (on this concern, see Olsson, 2002; Livingstone, 2004). As such, several studies on Internet's political significance tend to analyse the Internet in isolation from, rather than as a part of, the larger media environment. Finally, much of the research has taken a macro, overarching perspective of Internet and democracy, and not paid much attention to the Internet's significance in the context of the more concrete political engagement in everyday life. In what ways is the Internet really a resource to already politically engaged people's political activities? This chapter aims, in a modest way, to address these shortcomings.

Our research, using qualitative data from interviews with young citizens (15–19 years of age) who are politically active, has focused on their use of the traditional media as well as the Internet as resources for their role and identity as citizens. We have dealt with two categories of these young citizens, comprised of about two dozen respondents each. On the one hand are those who are involved in the youth organizations of the established political parties (Olsson, 2004), and on the other, those who are engaged in the so-called 'new politics' outside the party structure, often coloured by a focus on single issues or themes (Olsson, 2005b). Specifically, the extra-parliamentarian groups consist of Green Globalisation (an alter globalisation movement) and Friends of the Animals (an animal rights movement). In this chapter we deal largely with the second group, but summarise our findings from the first group to serve as a point of comparison.

The project has as a theoretical horizon, the notion of civic cultures that we have been developing, where such concepts as civic identities and practices have been used as an analytic frame (see Dahlgren, 2003, 2005, 2007; Dahlgren and Olsson, 2007). In this analytic framework, civic identity is understood as a component of the late-modern, composite self. Civic identity can take many forms; there are many ways of enacting citizenship and 'doing democracy'. Some sense of civic identity is a precondition for engagement; it is the subjective side of formal citizenship, where one feels in some way empowered such that engagement is experienced as meaningful. Today, there are many factors contributing to a decline in democratic participation, and civic cultures are often seen as weak, and thereby not fostering people's identities as citizens. There is an extensive literature on the dilemmas of democracy and the decline in civic engagement, not least among the young, but our concerns here are with empirical examples of young people who are democratically active, and how they make use of the Internet for their political purposes.

The Internet as a resource for an alternative political identity

Our main point of departure is how the Internet serves a resource for alternative political identities, and how it is perceived in this respect compared to traditional media. Various aspects of human identity have already been studied within Internet research. It might even be one of the most crowded areas in the study of the new ICTs. We can note a number of interesting, mostly theoretical contributions from the early years of Internet research (Turkle, 1995; Porter, 1997; Holmes, 1997). For instance, early on Derek Foster (1997) discussed the extent to which the new, digital media could help in shaping new communities and thus become important to the construction of individual identities.

These, and several similar early studies of identity dimensions on the Internet have been both effectively summarised and criticised by Don Slater:

The very idea of approaching the new media in terms of a sharp distinction between the online and the offline has given research in this area a peculiar profile. . . . the Internet has posed the possibility of entirely new relationships and identities, constituted within new media, and in competition with ostensibly non mediated, older forms of relationships. In this respect, the new media have been studied less as media that are used within existing social relations and practices, and more as a new social space which constitutes relations and practices on its own. The research agenda from this pint of view focuses not on the characteristics and uses of these media as means of communication but rather on the kinds of social life and cultures that they are capable of sustaining.

(Slater, 2002: 533)

We share Slater's critical view of these studies of the Internet's contribution to the construction of identities – not least his criticism against their preference for studying the Internet identity in isolation, with few, if any, connections to real life identities. This chapter uses a different premise, analysing the Internet as a resource for already – off-line – established political identities.

The idea of, specifically, 'political' identity is also in need of some additional qualification. The above-mentioned take on identity does, of course, also include political dimensions. For instance, it pays special interest in how the new information and communication technology, with its virtual worlds and interactive form, contributes to creating new subjects, or subject positions. Donna Haraways' (1985) by now classic essay on the cyborg is one obvious early example of this thread in research, and these lines of thought have been continuously developed ever since (for example, Willson, 1997; articles in Jones, 1994, 1998). Our interest here, however, lies not in how the Internet contributes to the creation of new subject positions and thus new political identities, but rather in young people's view of themselves as politically active and – more specifically – politically active within two political movements in Sweden, Green Globalisation and Friends of the Animals. As such, we are looking at political identities primarily constituted offline and understand the Internet as a resource to the continuous construction of such already established political identities.

Alternative political movements have been present in Internet research for quite some time, and there have been a number of suggestions as to how the net could become a resource for such activities. It is today well known – perhaps even a cliché – that the Internet was important to the Mexican Zapatistas' revolution in the mid-1990s and that the Internet played a crucial role in the protests surrounding the WTO's Seattle summit in 1999 (Kahn and Kellner, 2004). Further, Manuel Castells has emphasised how the net plays a key role for contemporary social movements, stressing how they become a force in the so-called 'Network society' (Castells,

1997; jfr. Hassan, 2004). Nevertheless, little effort has been aimed at how members of various alternative political movements actually make use of the Internet and its significance for their alternative political identity. In addressing these questions, we also take into consideration the traditional mass media. Through comparisons between how the young members in alternative political movements use and perceive traditional media and the Internet, the significance of the net becomes clearer.

Alternative perception of the traditional news media

In the first part of our research, focusing on the use of the Internet by young people who are involved with the youth groups of the established political parties (Olsson, 2004), it became clear to us that parliamentarian youth groups made very explicit use of the Internet for a variety of functions, including internal coordination and internal debate. Aside from these 'horizontal' activities, they also used the net to a great extent as an extension of the traditional mass media. They are very adept at using the technology and they follow the established news media via these organisations' online sites. In fact, they often find it more expedient to follow the mass media on the Internet than in the traditional newspaper or broadcast form. These young citizens are thus using the net for monitoring mainstream politics, rarely looking at political expression that lies beyond the boundaries of the parliamentarian parties. In this sense it can be said that they are solidifying mainstream political identities; a number of them even say that they plan to continue with party politics in the years ahead.

If we turn to the young citizens in the alternative political movements, a rather different picture emerges. These young respondents are quite obviously not very fond of traditional news media. Asta is the first respondent to make that very clear. She is a 16-year-old member in the alter-globalisation group Green Globalisation. She is a middle-class girl from a Swedish urban area. Just like the rest of the members in her organization, she pays special interest in issues of global, economic solidarity and ecological development. From these horizons she evaluates traditional news media:

Interviewer: I get kind of curious here. You don't use traditional media very much . . . but still you seem to hold a great deal of opinions . . . What inspires you?

Asta: Well, I get to hear quite a lot in the Internet discussions within Green Globalisation and in school and so on. The big issues . . . You get to know them anyway . . . but our issues [Green Globalisation] you don't really get through the news [ironic tone]. I don't know, but it feels like the [traditional] news media doesn't have much to say about them.

Interviewer: What do they do wrong then?

Asta: Well, not too many people share our interest in these issues. Hence, the news media pass them by. They don't fit with how they [the traditional news media] are used to describe the world. They perhaps think that our ideas are a bit too ideological.

Asta's colleagues within Green Globalisation are just as critical towards traditional news media as Asta is in this extract. To put it simply, they are quite dissatisfied with traditional news media's way of dealing with the issues that concern them. In the extract Asta explicitly criticises the weak representation afforded these issues within traditional news media, but she also – at least implicitly – touches upon a critique towards their market logic, that an issue has to attract a large audience in order to become 'news', and that Green Globalisation's position on these questions hardly qualify as such. They simply just do not attract a large enough audience to become news items within traditional media. As a consequence, she and her friends within Green Globalisation turn their back on them.

A similar view of traditional news media can be recognised in the interviews with the members of Friends of the Animals. Anna is 18 years old and currently finishing her last year in high school. She became a member of the organisation after taking the decision to become a vegetarian, and at this point she has been a member for three years. She lives in an urban area. At a stage in the interview she is asked to reflect upon where she finds news that is valuable to her and her friends within the organisation, and her reflections end in a critical view of traditional media's way of prioritising news in general, and paying attention to 'her' issues in particular:

Interviewer: Where do you find news that is valuable to you [and your political ideas]?
Anna: Hmmm . . . Mainly on mailing lists. On those lists people collect relevant news from their local papers and send them to the rest of us. . . . And . . . sometimes on the local pages in the newspaper, I check them to see if anything has happened locally.
Interviewer: What could that be? What's good to know?
Anna: I don't know . . . But in case something has happened . . . Well . . . I don't know . . . In case . . . But sometimes – not too often though – there is something interesting to read. But if there's something, I find it on the local pages, rarely on the pages for domestic or international news, since our news [news of interest to members of Friends of the Animals] isn't considered interesting enough. But on the local pages in the newspaper they sometimes report about demonstrations and actions. You rarely get that on national TV or radio. Instead it's sometimes on the local pages in the newspaper . . . or on the Internet.

It is primarily on mailing lists that Anna can find news important to her as a member of Friends of the Animals. On the Internet, various members collect information and distribute it to their colleagues. In terms of the traditional news media as news sources, they use mainly various local papers. In the local papers their organisation's whereabouts are at least, every once in a while, given some attention to. In general, though, Friends of the Animals is largely ignored. But on national TV and radio it is even worse: their organisation is never covered.

There is also another side to the criticism towards traditional news media among the members in these alternative political movements. Their critical points of view do not only deal with lack of representation. They are also about how they are represented on the few occasions where these issues are actually taken up. The issues are, they perceive, typically negatively angled and their organisations are framed as deviant.

Such views of traditional news media are made very clear in the interview with Gina, 15. She has been a member of Friends of the Animals for about a year. She lives in the same urban area and in this extract she makes her view of traditional news media very obvious:

Interviewer: Okay ... What do you mean about 'boring as hell' [...] when you talk about TV?

Gina: Like once ... there was this debate between a [member of Friends of the Animals] and a guy breeding minks. And it was all kind of angled to his disadvantage and I find that awfully sad.

[...]

Interviewer: Newspapers then, what about them?

Gina: [I dislike] how they present things, like they did about the attacks on the fur shop. This was last autumn, and I think the shop had, like, its thirtieth attack, and the newspapers went: 'This was made by militant vegans.' Then they just mention in passing that the attack was made by a very specific organisation, having nothing to do with us, but we end up getting blamed for these things even though we don't participate in them. I think that's very bad. Thanks to them we get a bad reputation and people become sceptical. But we're legal and stick to legal actions, we don't do these things, but the news media is misleading people.

Even though the two parts of the extract deals with different things – the first part with TV and the latter part with newspapers – they have one theme in common: how Friends of the Animals and affiliated organisations are represented in news media. In the first part, Gina criticises a specific TV news item in which a member of her organisation was framed as a deviant voice and their counterparts – a man representing the fur business – was represented as the voice of common sense. Thus, Friends of the Animals became 'the bad guys' and the fur business the 'good guys'. In the second part of the extract Gina addresses how the newspapers fail to correctly describe which organisations that engaged in illegal activism. Therefore, Gina's organisation – which adheres to legal actions, she says

– is unjustly blamed for these attacks. The news media simply put all animal right's activists into one and the same category of 'illegal' activists, without making much effort to distinguish between various groups. Gina is not alone in these views: most of those interviewed within Friends of the Animals as well as those in Green Globalisation share this view of the traditional media. They are certainly not happy about the way that the media tends to overlook their issues. These media are obviously not a very useful resource for their alternative political identities.

Alternative perception of the Internet

The Internet, however, is perceived in a completely different way among the young activists of the alternative organisations. Contrary to how traditional news media is perceived, the Internet is understood as a resource to their alternative political identities. 'On the Internet you find anything that you might need', Asta – a member of Green Globalisation – stresses, and her friends within the organisation (Rita and Sara) agree with her. On the Internet they find several resources for their alternative political identity and one passage from the interview with Rita (16) who lives in a major urban area, makes this especially obvious:

Interviewer: I thought . . . When it comes to your ideas about what political issues are important . . . Don't the media pay attention to them, at least every now and then? And doesn't that interest you?

Rita: Well, yes of course they do. That's what I read in the papers and what I watch when I watch TV. However . . . There are several sites on the Internet that I can visit instead, where I can meet people with an interest in my issues. You can talk [sic.] to people and you get to know about upcoming actions . . . and . . . I guess that's what I'm looking for.

Interviewer: You seem to select rather carefully . . .

Rita: Yes, I think so. You easily get influenced . . . so very influenced by what you see on TV. You take what you see for granted. And there's just so much shit, so I try to stay critical. But then . . . Neither do I have time to watch TV too much. . . . I've got more important things to do.

Rita starts the extract by once again asserting that traditional news media are useful in only a very limited way, and that she just picks very specific parts from what they have to offer. Instead, she understands the Internet to be a much more important resource. On the Internet she can find information that supports her alternative identity, and she also can meet and interact with people that are similar to herself.

The fact that the Internet is perceived as important for alternative political identities becomes even more obvious among the interviewees from Friends of the Animals. It is perhaps due to the fact that their political agenda breaks radically with mainstream politics and ideologies and that they, are therefore, in even more obvious need of alternative information. A very illustrative example is brought from the interview with Anna:

Interviewer: You mentioned a web site earlier . . . Vegan.nu . . . What's that?

Anna: That's a community, it's all about animal rights.

Interviewer: Have you been a member for a long time?

Anna: Well . . . Yes, I have. I became a member rather immediately after deciding to become a vegetarian. Someone recommended it to me. However, I don't participate too actively there, but they have a database for recipes and then I communicate with people.

Interviewer: What else is there?

Anna: You can discuss things . . . There's also news – on the first page – and then also . . . links to other web pages. Then you can buy and sell things there, like newspapers and books.

Through the Internet Anna and her friends within Friends of the Animals can get what they feel is relevant information, not least on the web community vegan.nu, where they can obtain news of interest to their alternative identity, discuss topics related to animal rights and meet with other animal rights activists. All in all, the community offers them a great deal of opportunity to continuously construct and reaffirm their sense of themselves as political actors with a decidedly alternative orientation. They can also get help for activities which lean more towards everyday cultural practices (recipes) rather than just explicitly political activities, which must be seen as contributing a sense of collective affinity. Thus, while traditional news media are perceived as hardly paying attention to the political issues these activists feel are important, or representing them in negative ways when they are covered, the Internet looms as a useful resource for both information and identity building.

Alternative uses of the Internet

Yet, more specifically, how do they actually make us of the Internet? Here we take a closer look at some of the practices that members of Green Globalisation and Friends of the Animals engage in through the net. Green Globalisation members are by no means typical computer 'nerds', but they readily underscore its importance. First of all they are careful to make it clear that the Internet is used as a resource for internal coordination within the organisation. Asta, who holds an important position within the organisation on the local level, carefully describes how she and her colleagues use the net for local mailing lists. Through these lists local members distribute information to one another about, for instance, calls for meetings and current activities. Next, she also relates how the organ-isation uses regional mailing lists, which contain more general information about the organisation's activities at this level. On the regional level the organisation is also involved in web publishing, and they use these web pages for both internal (within Green Globalisation) and external (with the wider public) communication about the organisation's ideas and activities. Turning to the national level, the organisation also uses mailing lists and has a national web page presenting Green Globalisation to the wider public, in the hope of attracting new members.

Apart from these uses, the Internet is also used in a informal manner within Green Globalisation. In the interview Asta describes how various informal networks within the organisation are shaped through the Internet. In these networks members with similar special interests meet one another in mutual discussions and/or get-togethers. For example, Asta mentions the feminist network and the woodworking crafts network. These networks exclusively involve members of the organisation, but they do not follow the organisation's formal structures. Hence, they are web-based informal networks within the formal organisation.

Another member of Green Globalisation, Sara (16), who lives in the countryside nearby a Swedish city, comes from a small local group that does not make much use of the Internet for internal coordination. However, she does make use of the Internet in other ways. In the interview she explains how lately the net has become helpful in terms of everyday activism:

Sara: [We're into] ad-busting, that's something new, where we . . . You know . . . unethical commercials . . . We collect information about the company in question in order to make sure that we're right to criticise them. Then we've – if it is perhaps sexist commercials – balloons that say: 'You can't buy me', that we put on the ads. Or: 'The ad has been taken away due to its unethical message.'

[. . .]

Interviewer: What's the name of the web site?

Sara: Adsabotage.org (in Swedish: reklamsabotage.org) . . . But you have to be careful, you need to check your facts before you move on to action. If you get it wrong it'll be destructive for the whole organisation.

Interviewer: How does it work?

Sara: They've got . . . They've for instance . . . You can order and then print these balloons and they also have instructions about how you can go about. But we're careful not to destroy anything. We're only trying to make people open their eyes.

In this latest addition to Sara's repertoire of everyday activism – the 'culture-jamming' of ads – she and her activist friends subvert what they see as unethical commercials by altering the messages. In this practice the Internet is an indispensable resource. On websites such as reklamsabotage.org – which is a kind of Swedish equivalence to the internationally famous adbusters.org – she and her friends find the necessary material to this destruction: stickers with pre-printed alternative messages, models for posters and also a gallery to inspire the creation of alternative messages. At they same time, the net is used to research the targeted corporation so the activists can be sure that the allegation of lack of ethics is correct, before proceeding to subvert the advertisements.

Turning to Friends of the Animals, Emma, who is 18 years old and lives in the countryside nearby a city, describes how she uses the Internet in order to maintain her personal contacts within the organisation and to keep herself up to date with its developments. Several times a day she receives emails from her local organisation as well as the nationwide organisation. In Emma's case these emails are also her main contact with the organisation, since her local group does not have many face-to-face meetings.

Anna relates a similar use of the Internet. Even though her face-to-face activities within Friends of the Animals are more frequent than Emma's, many of her contacts with the organization are also web-based:

Interviewer: Are there other websites that you usually visit?
Anna: Well, not that I visit in order to check up on things . . . But usually I visit our websites [Friends of the Animals] quite a lot and then I also get emails from the mailing lists quite often.
[. . .]
Interviewer: Tell me more about these lists . . .
Anna: It's also . . . if you find something that might be of interest to other members you mail it there. And then it's also good for quick dissemination of information within the organisation. And if you have a piece of news it's an easy way of sharing it with other members.

Initially Anna repeats Emma's statement about these lists, that they are used for internal coordination. She also mentions frequent visits to the organisation's websites as an important web practice. More interesting though is her description of how she and other subscribers to the mailing lists use them to disseminate news to one another. Especially interesting is perhaps the fact that the news, Anna explains, not only deals with the organisation's internal affairs, but also updates on what is happening in the world outside the organisation that is of relevance. Gina also discusses this kind of updating, and she is more concrete in terms of the kind of news that is posted on these lists: 'It can be something about new rules and regulations for the food industry, perhaps new regulations of how big the cages that keep chickens must be.' Arguably, for these members of Friends of the Animals, the Internet provides them with important continual monitoring of the external environment as well with a means for keeping abreast of the organisation itself.

The fact that the Internet is, in various ways, an important tool for the members in Friends of the Animals makes it somewhat surprising to see Gina claim that she does not engage in any discussions on the net:

Interviewer: What do you do on the Internet?

Gina: I check my mails . . . I mostly get mails from Friends of the Animals, like protocols and stuff – like instructions about where to meet and what I'm supposed to do and information about coming events. But also things that'll happen later on.

[. . .]

Interviewer: The mails you receive . . . Do you engage in discussions over the Internet?

Gina: No, we're all of the same opinion so we don't discuss anything.

It appears that she does not really understand the essence of discussion, that they can be valuable even among people who share the same point of view. However, after thinking the issue through for a while she realises that she actually has seen a lot of discussions taking place on the Internet in connection with Friends of the Animals:

Gina: But wait a minute . . . Just before Christmas we had a discussion on how to carry an action through.

Her friends within Friends of the Animals are more familiar with the frequent debates and discussions on the net that do take place between members of Friends of the Animals. Emma certainly seems to be a frequent reader of these debates as well as a quite experienced participator:

Interviewer: You seem to discuss pretty hands on questions . . . Don't you ever move into ideological debates [on the Internet]?

Emma: Yes we do . . . Sometimes we do . . . A lot of these . . . There are subsections [in the debate] so you can discuss different things, not only hands on things. We also discuss different points of view.

Interviewer: Do you participate in these discussions?

Emma: I mostly read them, I think.

Interviewer: What do you write, then, when you participate?

Emma: I usually discuss . . . try to make decisions about what we should do and how.

Interviewer: Is there a discussion?

Emma: Yes, if someone has an idea about something we do that. We discuss how things can be done.

It is quite obvious that Emma knows her ways around the debates on the Internet. She makes an initiated description of it, that it takes place on various levels within the organisation, and that everything from day-today matters to ideological questions are brought up. She also participates in these debates, mostly when it comes to hands-on issues, but she is also a close reader when ideological topics arise. However, Emma does not tell us a lot about what kinds of ideological issues are brought up, but on that matter Anna – her colleague within Friends of the Animals – offers a more concrete example:

Interviewer: What do you discuss on the Internet?
Anna: Well . . . It's things like . . . It was in the local paper the other day . . . The fur shop . . . they had . . . There was a window that already was broken by one group of activists and then another group of activists later on filled the shop with foam from a fire extinguisher. Then some people thought it was a bad idea to do that, since it's well known that the owner usually sleeps in his shop and that he might get physically hurt. But some other people thought that it was all right to do so . . . Most often it has to do with what actions are OK and what actions aren't.

Anna describes what the debate can look like and what subjects are brought up for discussion. She picks a recent example, a debate between members of Friends of the Animals that dealt with that kinds of actions that the organisation should consider as legitimate or illegitimate. From her description we can see that the debate even touches on moral and ethical values as the discussion delves into questions such as what actions should be considered legitimate in the efforts to support the animals' rights. These discussions are rather frequent, Anna says, but she also – like Emma – points to the fact that discussions have a more concrete character, dealing with issues of internal coordination.

All in all, it is obvious that the interviewees from Friends of the Animals make good use of the Internet in their political efforts. They use it as a tool for internal coordination, like calling for meetings and informing about coming actions. Furthermore, it appears to be an important source for alternative information, especially as the mailing lists are used to distribute news from all over the world. Finally, they also use it as an internal public sphere where everything from forthcoming actions to moral values are dealt with.

Conclusion

As it has been shown in the initial sections, this chapter draws inspiration from two established areas in Internet research. On the one hand research on the Internet and identity, and on the other hand research on Internet's practical significance for alternative political movements. From that point of departure it has aimed at partially integrating the areas in an analysis of the use and perception of the Internet, as well as traditional news media, among young citizens that are active within alternative political movements.

With regard to research into the Internet's significance for identity construction – the chapter moves away from the dominant preference for understanding Internet-related identity construction as an isolated phenomenon, taking place exclusively on the Internet. Instead, the chapter understands the Internet as a resource contributing to the continuous construction of already (mainly offline) established identities and more specifically political identities. Hence, it argues for a contextualisation of the Internet users.

With reference to research into the Internet's significance for alternative political movements, this chapter has first aimed to provide empirical illustrations of how the Internet is used by young people with an alternative political identity. There are, therefore, several empirical illustrations of various Internet practices conducted by young, active citizens. Second, it has also started to test a new approach to research in this area by focusing on members' political identities.

We have seen how the Internet has been shaped into an important resource by young respondents as a support for their alternative political identity. All respondents agree on the Internet's value to them as members of alternative political organisations. In comparison with how traditional news media are perceived, it is especially true that the Internet offers them something that other media do not. The Internet provides, among other things, alternative information, internal coordination, contacts with like-minded people, access to public spheres beyond the organisation, and a resource for everyday activism.

Last, there is the methodological question about contextualising the Internet as one of several media in people's everyday lives. Most studies tend to focus quite exclusively on the Internet, but in attempting to understand the significance of the net (or any other everyday medium), we should carefully situate the given medium within a larger media environment that people have access to and in which they operate. As such, the uses to which any given medium is put, as well as the perceptions of it, could be more easily understood, and analysed, if we consider how it relates to other media that people use. In the analysis conducted here, we have made comparative use of the respondents' perception and use of traditional news media in illuminating the significance the Internet has for them.

Whether or not this methodological recommendation is useful will vary depending on the research project at hand, but we would generally posit that in looking at the Internet in terms of people's everyday lives, consideration of the other media to which the respondents avail themselves will help to deepen the analysis. Comparisons can help to illuminate what is special about the Internet compared to other, traditional media. But in other contexts, this methodological approach can also help prevent overestimating the net's significance (Olsson, 2002; Olsson, 2006), which has sometimes been the case within Internet research. Given the rapid technological developments and convergences at work in the media landscape, we must be increasingly alert to what 'Internet' exactly means; with many of the traditional mass media having moved onto the net, the specificity of what we mean by 'the net' or 'the web' becomes increasing problematic.

6 Youth online

Researching the political use of the Internet in the Italian context[1]

Davide Calenda and Lorenzo Mosca

Introduction: young people and politics in the Italian context

Between the end of the 1980s and the beginning of the last decade different phenomena (at both national and international levels) gave rise to significant changes in Italy. The post-war political system (characterised by a blocked political system excluding the Communist party from the government) collapsed, and a new bipolar party system, based on competition between two coalitions (centre-left and centre-right) arose. Yet in recent times many factors combined have contributed to a decline in trust among citizens towards national politics, political parties and institutions in Italy (Mannheimer and Sani, 2001). These factors include the weakening of ideology following the fall of the Berlin wall, the increasing importance of international politics in national arenas (due to increased financial and economic globalisation, as well as European integration), and, finally, in relation to the Italian system, political corruption scandals (Mantovani and Burnett, 1998).

Studies on the attitudes of young Italians in the 1990s highlighted an increasing lack of interest in politics (Cavalli and De Lillo, 1993), with significant mistrust in political parties and institutions (Cartocci, 2002). That said, other studies have underlined a strong politicisation among the generation aged 18 to 24 during this same period, characterised by an increasing interest in politics and a general orientation towards the left side of the political spectrum, in comparison with older generations. Within the same cohort a difference concerning the values and political orientations of students and non-students was observed. While students tended to be more left-wing, non-students were found to hold more right-wing tendencies (Cartocci and Corbetta, 2001). Furthermore, multiple similarities have been underlined between the generations politically socialised between 1968 and 1977 (a period of strong social uprisings in Italy) and those aged between 18 and 24 socialised during the 1990s (see the Italian National Elections Studies – ITANES – 2001).

A recent survey on political participation among young people aged 15 to 25 in eight European countries (EUYOUPART, 2005) has shown that the majority of the 8,030 people interviewed were not very interested in politics, mistrusting traditional political actors, yet also displaying idealistic and polarised views of politics.

Turning to Italy in particular, the general situation is characterised by three important aspects. First, there is an high degree of politicisation in the Italian context. Close-knit families and friendships facilitate the political socialisation of young people (EUYOUPART 2005: 94–6).

Second, young people express positive attitudes towards participation. Eighty-five per cent had voted in elections, compared with an average turnout of approximately 50 per cent in the other countries included in the survey (ibid.: 24–9), while 49 per cent participated in demonstrations, and 28 per cent in the occupation of public or private buildings. Participation in civil society organisations was also fairly widely diffused – 10 per cent were involved in pacifist organisations, 15 per cent in charities, 20 per cent in religious organisations, 21 per cent in youth organisations, and 24 per cent in cultural organisations. At the same time, involvement in traditional political organisations was very limited. Only 4 per cent were members of youth party organisations, 3 per cent of political parties and just 2 per cent adhered to trade unions. Third, mistrust in the political system and especially in politicians was shown to be widely shared among young people.

Only 11 per cent of all the Italian respondents trusted political parties, 59 per cent did not, and 30 per cent were indifferent. It is also worth noting that politicians gained a very low score on trust among young Italian people (7 per cent). In fact, as the authors note, 'this is the item with the relatively least indifference (20 per cent), which means a very high overall distrust' (ibid.: 41–5). Trust is instead invested, for the most part, in civil society organisations such as Amnesty International (55 per cent), while 30 per cent declared themselves in favour of the movement against neo-liberal globalisation, although direct participation in anti-globalisation associations is not high (see the Italian Report, Cornolti *et al.*, 2005; for a more detailed analysis, see Bontempi and Pocaterra, 2007).

Italian young people see politics as something positive: political activism is a means 'to build a better world' for 91 per cent of the sample (ibid.: 10). In addition, Italian young people score highest, in comparison with the young people from other countries interviewed, in thinking that participating in NGOs represents an effective form of political participation.

These data, although more in-depth analysis is needed, do provide some support for the hypothesis that political participation is undergoing something of a resurrection amongst Italian youth. Norris talks of 'a phoenix rising from the ashes', referring to the fact that disengagement from traditional, conventional and 'old' forms of participation appears to have created new resources that feed on innovative, unconventional and 'new' forms (Norris, 2002). Our contribution assesses the relationships between different forms of political participation and the use of the Internet. The analysis is based on two surveys of Italian students with experience of 'old' and 'new' forms of participation. The main question addressed is *whether* and *how* the political characteristics of students (political orientation, organisational participation and political action)[2] influence the way they use the Internet for political purposes.

In the first part of the chapter, we present the two different pieces of research on Italian students. A synthetic review of the central aspects of the debate around the implications of the Internet for political participation follows. We then move on to present some empirical results: describing, first, the demographic features of students included in our samples and their political orientations. We then address the relationships between their political characteristics and their political use of the Internet. Finally, the main results from these two studies are discussed.

Characteristics of the research

The first survey was carried out in 2001 (September–November) through a web questionnaire addressed to students at the University of Florence (UF). The second was carried out in November 2002 and addressed participants of the European Social Forum (ESF) in Florence. Both were developed through the self-administration of a structured questionnaire.[3] While the two questionnaires were designed for two different studies, they did share common indicators of political participation and Internet use.

The UF survey is based on a self-selected sample and is thus unrepresentative of the student population as a whole. However, sample characteristics are fairly coherent with the general demographic characteristics of the student population for the years 2000–01.[4] Concerning the survey of ESF participants, here the research design was developed in order to work with a 'non-probabilistic sample' (Corbetta, 1999: 343–52).[5] The sampling strategy was based on previous studies on social movements in Italy (della Porta, 1996; Andretta *et al.*, 2002). The survey was implemented using a 'strategy of small samples', focusing on the main organisational sectors of the Italian movement, mapping their presence in the ESF (with reference to the official programme) and then randomly selecting interviewees during the main events organised by the different movement sectors. Therefore, we used a sampling method of selecting interviewees on the basis of their membership of organisational sectors (for more details see della Porta *et al.*, 2006). In order to allow for better comparisons between the two samples, and in line with the objective of analysing the links between the Internet and political participation, case selection was based on the following criteria. Within the UF sample, we selected only those students who had participated in (or had stated they were likely to participate in) a demonstration on globalization issues.[6] Within the ESF sample, we selected only those students belonging to different Italian universities and using the

Internet at least once a month.[7] On the basis of these criteria we obtained a sample of 880 cases, from which we randomly extracted 200 cases in order to build a sample of a similar size to the UF study.

Considering that the non-probabilistic nature of our samples does not allow strong inferences to be made, we decided to use descriptive statistics and non-parametric correlations in order to give an idea of the strength of the relations between variables.[8] For some of the cases, in order to make our results more intelligible, we used synthetic indexes created by aggregating various indicators. This applies to the indexes of political action,[9] organisational participation,[10] and political use of the Internet.[11]

The Internet for participation: a brief overview of limits and opportunities

Regarding online political participation, one important aspect to be considered is the level of Internet access. McChesney (1996), for example, has spoken of a 'partial' public sphere in cyberspace, due to the fact that Internet access is still very much limited to well-educated people with high incomes, while female and older persons generally have lower rates of access. Even if Internet access has widened in the past decade, European statistics on Internet diffusion in the last five years indicate that southern European countries have lower levels of penetration as compared to northern European countries (Eurobarometer, 2000; Eurostat, 2005a).

On the causes of this European digital divide, Eurobarometer indicated that, although 'the use of each technology appears to follow varied patterns among social-demographic groups ... gender is, on average, the least discriminating variable, while countries, income and education are the most significant sources of disparities' (2000: 16–17). However, when we look at the differences among European countries, we notice that gender inequalities in Internet access apply mainly to southern Europe. Concerning age, the most 'connected' people fall into the 16 to 24 age category in all European countries (Eurostat, 2005a). A survey carried out in Italy in 2001 showed similar trends (Censis, 2001). Indeed, from 2002 to 2005 the percentage of households with Internet access in Italy has always fallen below the average in old member states (EU15). Household connections have grown from 34 to 39 per cent in Italy and from 39 to 53 per cent in the EU15 (Eurostat, 2005b).

Similar trends apply to broadband penetration rates. A difference in Internet use between social sectors with different degrees of interest in politics also exists: the medium is most used for political purposes by citizens already active and interested in politics (Norris, 2001: 238). The EUYOUPART study (2005) for instance, found that the use of the Internet among young people to find out and discuss politics is always associated with high levels of interest and participation.

However, the progressive integration of the Internet into the everyday life of people and organisations has led to a widening of scholarly attention to cyberspace as a 'playground' of political participation (van de Donk *et al.*, 2004; della Porta and Mosca, 2005) providing opportunities for social and political engagement (Castells, 1996). Analyses vary from focusing on individual attitudes (for example, Katz *et al.*, 2001; Wellman and Haythornthwaite, 2002) to the use of the Internet by social and political groups (for example, for environmental movements, see Dordoy and Mellor, 2001; Pickerill, 2003; for NGOs, see Warkentin, 2001; for feminists, see Ayers, 2003; for social movements, see van de Donk *et al.*, 2004: part III; della Porta *et al.*, 2006).

Analyses focusing on individuals have mainly addressed the associations between Internet use and civic engagement. In the United States for instance, scholars have attempted to answer the question of whether the Internet could slow down the progressive decline in citizens' engagement, as depicted by some authors (see Putnam, 2000).

The results of the more recent Internet studies led most scholars to agree that the Internet does not reduce social and political engagement (see for instance the debate developed in Wellman and Haythornthwaite, 2002). Indeed, it has been noted that frequent Internet use 'is associated with high participatory involvement in organizations and politics' and 'online political discussion appears to be an extension of offline activity' (Wellman *et al.*, 2001: 448). In general terms, a picture of a 'supplementary' effect of the Internet on civic engagement and political participation has been drawn. Haythornthwaite and Wellman have pointed out that the Internet 'does not function on its own, but is embedded in the real life things that people do' (Haythornthwaite and Wellman, 2002: 7). As with any other technology (MacKenzie and Wajcman, 1985; Williams and Edge, 1996; Dutton, 2005), the development and use of the Internet can be seen as social processes. The Internet is shaped by people but, at the same time, the technology influences the patterns of everyday life in specific ways (see Castells 2001, Chapter 5).

This chapter is intended to contribute to this discussion by focusing on how the political characteristics of students may shape the use of the Internet for political purposes. We understand that this is only one side of the question, but at this stage of the research it is not possible to provide empirical evidence of how the medium itself shapes political behaviours. First, we explore whether people already engaged offline will also use the Internet for political purposes. Second, we consider different forms of offline engagement, specifically organisational participation and political action. We then analyse whether these forms of participation have an influence on the political use of the Internet.

Demographic characteristics of students and political engagement

The samples on which this study is based are composed of well-educated young people. This means that the analysis focuses on a specific group in society which should not display great inequalities in terms of Internet access. However, in line with the general trends of Internet use in Italy as described above, we found gender differences in time spent on the Internet within our samples. Although the difference was not statistically significant in the UF sample, in the ESF sample we found a clear, but not dramatic, variation.[12] The gender divide in the ESF sample is also reflected in the political use of the Internet: the non-parametric test for two independent samples (Mann-Whitney U Test) reports a significant difference (Z –3.106**). However, no gender differences were found when considering organisational participation and political action.[13]

A similar situation is found in relation to age, which influences time spent on the Internet for students from both samples. In the UF sample age is significantly correlated with time spent online (0.216**) while in the ESF sample the correlation is somewhat lower (0.157**).

As with gender, age is not significantly associated with the indexes of organisational participation and political action.

However, age differences as related to time spent on the Internet are also reproduced with regard to the political use of the medium. In the two samples age is correlated with the index of political use of the Internet (0.181** in the UF sample; 0.172** in the ESF sample). To summarise, the trend we observed indicates that time spent on the Internet, which varies according to gender and age, matters when we take into account the index of political use of the Internet. In this case the Internet reinforces the political participation of people already engaged offline, who spend the most time online.

Nonetheless, we found that gender and age inequalities regarding time spent online could not explain how the Internet is used for different purposes: information, communication or action. As will be seen in the following sections, the political characteristics of students allow us to shed light on different styles of online participation.

Political orientation and participation

It is worth reiterating that the findings used in this chapter focus on young people involved in, or at least close to, movements mobilising around globalisation issues. Consequently, only a small part of the political spectrum is embraced by our analysis.[14] Before focusing on the political use of the Internet by the students in our samples, we present the main findings concerning the relationships between political orientation and political participation. This decision is based on the fact that we hypothesise that both these dimensions may shape the ways in which the Internet is used for political participation.[15]

As Table 6.1 shows, the degrees of organisational participation and political action in the UF sample are lower than in the ESF sample. It is

Table 6.1 Political characteristics of students

	ESF (%)	UF (%)
Type of organisational participation (at least one)		
Political party and trade unions	31.2	8.1
Voluntary/charity, NGO, religious	66.8	28.4
Other civil society organisations	81.5	18.8
Total (N)	**195–199**	**197**
Type of non-organisational participation (at least one)		
Non-radical	100.0	77.2
Radical	23.2	8.6
Total (N)	**193–198**	**197**

also worth noting that ESF students are more likely than UF students to have experienced multiple organisational affiliations. In the ESF sample, all interviewees had participated in at least one form of political action (whether radical or non-radical),[16] compared with 78.2 per cent in the UF sample. Some 97 per cent of students in the ESF sample had participated in at least one organisation, against 51.8 per cent in the UF sample.[17]

In both samples, although participation in traditional political organisations is present, most of the students tend to devote themselves to engagement in civil society organisations, especially voluntary/charity organisations, NGOs and religious groups.[18]

Our data show that political participation is associated with political orientation. In the UF sample we observed that engagement in political action (synthetic index) increases as we move to the left side of the political spectrum (0.297**).[19] This is the case, for instance, not only for the categories 'active in a political party' (0.240**) and 'support electoral campaign' (0.221**), but also for participation in radical forms of political action such as 'disruptive demonstrations' (0.198**) and 'occupying abandoned buildings' (0.199**).

In the ESF sample we found similar trends: political orientation and political action (synthetic index) are significantly correlated (0.337**). More specifically, political orientation is related to different forms of action like striking (0.185**), boycotting (0.226**), sit-ins (0.251**), leafleting (0.271**), occupying abandoned buildings (0.350**) and violence against property (0.271**).

In the following section, we turn our focus to a factor more usually ignored by surveys on Internet usage: the influence of political characteristics on Internet use.

Political characteristics of students and their influence on the political use of the Internet

The Internet can be seen as a resource that supports political participation in several ways: by providing a new platform for information retrieval, debate and engagement; or by complementing offline participation by, for instance, facilitating the flow of information and communication between people already involved in social and political networks.

This section is intended to contribute to this discussion by focusing on one main research question. We attempt to answer the question of just how the relationship between offline and online participation works, that is, if, and how, the political use of the Internet is shaped by young people according to their political characteristics. First, we stress the fact that offline and online participation are associated. The index of the political use of the Internet is correlated with organisational participation in both samples (0.327** in the ESF; 0.209** in the UF). The importance of organisational participation is confirmed in both studies when we analyse the association between participation in an organisation that uses the Internet and the index of the political use of the Internet (0.349** in the ESF; 0.178** in the UF).

Regarding the correlation between the political use of the Internet and the index of political action, this is significant only in the ESF sample (0.364**). This difference is explained by the fact that within the ESF sample, many students have experiences in both kinds of participation (0.366**), while in the UF case this correlation is not significant. However, it is worth noting that if in the UF sample we select only those students who declared they had participated in a demonstration on globalisation issues, similar trends highlighted by the ESF research are found concerning the political use of the Internet.[20]

We now turn to our research question. Table 6.2 shows the indicators of political use of the Internet that were included in both studies, and on which we focus most of the comparative analysis.

The table shows some differences that must be interpreted by considering the different features of the two samples. As we have already underlined, the ESF sample includes students engaged in social movements characterised

Table 6.2 Different types of political use of the Internet

Types of political use of the Internet	ESF (%)	UF (%)
Retrieving alternative information	82.4	31.0
Debating online	47.2	45.7
Petitioning/campaigning online	59.2	50.3
Net-striking	15.9	2.0
Total (N)	**193–197**	**197**

by their intense use of the Internet to organise and carry out political actions. The issues around which they mobilise are scarcely considered by the traditional mass media, and are underrepresented in parliamentary arenas. Consequently, the Internet is heavily used both as an alternative medium and as a means for protest. Interestingly, debating and campaigning online are similarly distributed in both samples. This may indicate that these activities are not strongly associated with strictly political characteristics.

Regarding information, no trade-off between online and offline information consumption emerges in our data. However, some differences were found concerning the political characteristics of students. We included, in both studies, indicators regarding both online information access and the types of information retrieved online during two specific political events: the 2001 Italian general elections, and the 2002 European Social Forum in Florence.

In the UF sample, the Internet was most used during the 2001 general elections by students more involved in traditional forms of political participation (those classified as non-radical in Table 6.1). The correlation between the index of non-radical political action and use of the Internet for retrieving information during the electoral campaign is 0.293**. In the ESF sample the Internet was used both before and during the social forum for accessing information on the agenda and events by 75.3 per cent of students (the correlation with the index of political action is not significant). Regarding the type of information retrieved online, we focused on the Internet as an alternative source of information.

In the ESF sample, the data show that the Internet is used both to complement information available through the traditional media and to obtain information that cannot be found in the conventional public sphere. Moreover, mistrust of traditional media is positively correlated with the search for alternative information online (0.177**).[21] A strong relationship exists between having used the Internet in an organisation and using it to search for alternative information (0.443**). The need for organisations to collect as much information as possible in order to carry out their activities – including the online variety – leads their members to exploit the informative potential of the Internet.

In the UF sample, selecting only those students who have participated in a demonstration on globalisation issues, we find an attitude towards the Internet as an alternative means of information similar to that observed in the ESF sample (Chi Square Test: 4.054*).

Regarding communication, although our data do not allow us to make strong inferences about participation in online debates, the findings at least seem to indicate that, as Wellman has pointed out, 'rather than distinct online and offline spheres, people are using whatever means are appropriate and available at the moment to participate in organizations and politics. People already participating offline will use the Internet to augment and extend their participation' (Wellman *et al.*, 2001: 450).

Almost half of the students in both samples have expressed political opinions in forums and/or mailing lists. In the ESF sample, expressing political opinions online is correlated with both organisational participation (0.242**) and political action (0.307**). Furthermore, Internet use in an organisation is correlated with its use to express political opinions (0.288**). This data suggests that these students used the Internet to maintain existing ties within the social and political networks in which they take part. This is coherent with the general picture that describes social movement participants as very interested in using the Internet as a means for political debate (Andretta *et al.*, 2002).

In the UF sample debating in forums is not significantly influenced by participation in organisations.[22] However, if we look at single political indicators, we see that, similar to the trends observed in the ESF sample, online forums were mainly used by students with more radical political orientations, preoccupied with globalisation issues: among those who debated online, 61 per cent had participated in a demonstration on globalisation issues (0.191**), and 75 per cent were leftist students (the correlation between political orientation and debating online is 0.169*).

The lack of association between offline participation and online discussion may indicate that the Internet is seen by some students as a new platform for talking politics. In order to better explore this hypothesis, we built a typology combining different forms of offline participation. Four types of participation were identified: no participation; organisational participation only; political action only; and a final type incorporating both of the latter forms of participation. We then analysed how online discussion is distributed among the four types.

Interestingly, the group of students involved in organisations, but not in political action, scores lowest (20 per cent), while the group of those who do not participate at all and the group of those engaged only in political action display the same score (25.6 per cent). The group of those engaged in both forms of participation scores highest (28.9 per cent). These data seem to indicate that different patterns of Internet use for political discussion coexist. On the one hand, the Internet is an additional resource for participation for those more involved in politics; on the other, this medium also represents a means of participation for those less likely to be directly engaged in offline organisations and political action. The Internet has also been perceived as a medium providing a new chance for political action. The indicators of online action included in our studies referred to campaigning online and protesting online.

We included in the latter category electronic disturbance actions such as net-strikes (a form of online protest intended to 'jam' a website considered a symbolic target; see Jordan, 2002). In both of the samples, as shown above, the net-strike is rare: 15.9 per cent of respondents in the ESF sample have participated in such actions, and only 2 per cent in the UF sample.[23]

In the ESF sample net-striking is correlated with participation in sit-ins (0.210**), in boycotts (0.215**), in violent actions against property (0.225**) and with participation in social centres (0.199**). Hence, offline participation in unconventional and radical actions is reproduced online. This consistency between offline and online actions was also found for more moderate forms of action, such as participation in online campaigns. In both samples, we found that online campaigning is correlated with participation in voluntary or charitable organisations, NGOs and religious groups (0.239** in the ESF sample; 0.187** in the UF sample).[24] This may be explained by the fact that online campaigns mostly concern issues which match the cultural identities of these organisations. In the UF research we included several items regarding the type of issues that students supported through online campaigns. Human and civil rights issues scored highest (43.7 per cent) followed by solidarity (24 per cent) and environmental issues (21 per cent), critical issues related to the Internet (12 per cent), bio-ethical issues (6 per cent) and political issues (2 per cent).

Conclusion

The findings presented above indicate the presence of two, connected, relationships between offline and online participation. First, people already engaged in offline social and political networks use the Internet to consolidate their participation. Second, the data show that the general characteristics of offline participation among students are reproduced online.

Regarding the first point, we observed that the more our students are engaged in different social and political networks, the more they used the Internet to reinforce their participation. This seems to mirror the general observation of several scholars that a greater use of the Internet is associated with larger social (and political) networks (Di Maggio *et al.*, 2001: 316).

However, the distinction we made between organisational participation and political action allowed us to explore in more depth the links between these types of participation and the political use of the Internet. Our data indicate that, although it has been noted that most political actions can be seen as organisational involvement (Wellman *et al.*, 2001: 447), the latter has a greater influence on online participation. We have observed that when the association between organisational participation and political action is less strong, as in the case of the UF sample, students who reported less participation in organisations also participate less online. The importance of organisational participation is confirmed by other findings. In particular, our data show that participating in 'wired' organisations is associated with the highest scores for Internet use for political purposes. The fact that both political and civil society organisations increasingly use the Internet to arrange their activities could well be important in explaining this trend. Regarding the second point, several findings lead us to suggest the hypothesis that there is consistency between online and offline practices of political participation. In fact, from our results it is evident that students tend to reproduce their offline styles of participation online. Consistency between offline and online styles of participation, albeit with some differences, exists regarding information, communication and action. Concerning the type of information retrieved online, students more engaged with globalisation issues tend to see the Internet as an alternative source of information.

The data on using the Internet for online debating indicate that this possibility is mainly exploited for practical reasons. From the analysis of the ESF data it emerged that online debating appeared to be used to consolidate existing offline ties and to support organisational participation through online 'endless assemblies'. Indeed, it has been observed that electronic networks are the backbone of new social movements (Castells, 2001: 142). Other authors have pointed out the usefulness of the Internet for facilitating flows of information in the periods between face-to-face meetings, and for arranging the meetings themselves (see Wellman and Haythornthwaite, 2002).

In the UF sample there is no statistically significant evidence that online debate is an extension of offline participation, except for more radical and engaged students, who generally display patterns of Internet usage similar to those of the students in the ESF sample. However, the fact that offline participation in the UF sample does not always explain students' engagement in online debates, suggests that the Internet may have been used by students as a new platform for talking politics. Finally, regarding online political action, we found consistency between offline and online actions for both moderate forms of engagement (online campaigns) and more radical forms (electronic disturbance action). For radical online forms of action in particular, the Internet seems to be used to bridge online and offline activism (see also Jordan, 2002).

To conclude, our data support the hypothesis of the social (political) shaping of the Internet. However, further research should focus on whether and how the Internet contributes to change political participation. As some scholars have claimed (see for instance Coleman and Rowe, 2005), the Internet may be seen by younger people as a more appropriate medium through which newer, more creative forms of communication and participation can take place.

Notes

1 Although the authors share responsibility for the whole chapter, David Calenda wrote the following paragraphs: Introduction; Characteristics of the research; Political characteristics of students and their influence on the political use of the Internet. Lorenzo Mosca wrote the following paragraphs: The Internet for participation; Demographic characteristics of students and political engagement; Political orientation and participation; Conclusion.

2 More details on the specific indicators will be specified in notes 9, 10 and 14.
3 In the UF research, the questionnaire was published on the University of Florence website, both on the home page and in the section specifically devoted to delivering services to students, and filled in online. Access was controlled through a log-in form. In the ESF research, data were collected through a self-administered paper-based questionnaire during the social forum.
4 In the UF sample females are slightly overrepresented in reference to the University of Florence population, while no differences were found concerning the average age. General statistics on the UF population can be found on the Italian Ministry of University and Research website (http://www.miur.it/ustat/default.asp).
5 A probabilistic sample could not be built, since there is no way of knowing the characteristics of the population participating in civil society events before they take place (indeed, lists of participants do not even exist).
6 Overall, 380 questionnaires were collected; among these 197 cases were selected for the purpose of the study presented here. Students who filled in the questionnaire belonged to different academic fields that can be summarised as follows: 49.7 per cent to social and economic sciences; 18.3 per cent to natural sciences and engineering; 17.8 per cent to humanities; 14.2 per cent to architecture. The choice to include both students who had actually participated (21 per cent) in a demonstration on globalisation issues as well as those who stated they might participate in the future (79 per cent), is based on the fact that when the survey was conducted the dramatic events of the anti-G8 demonstration in Genoa in July 2001 had just occurred and were fresh in people's minds. This led us to suppose that, given the emotionally-charged context of the period, declaring sympathy for these demonstrations represented a reliable indication of students' closeness to globalisation issues. We then checked the general political characteristics of this sample and observed that most of the students reported similar experiences of political participation, although with lower rates, as those of the ESF sample. We considered this difference a richness which allowed us to explore a wider spectrum of political characteristics in the comparative analysis.
7 For both samples the frequency of Internet use was operationalised as follows: 'one or two times a week or less frequently' (27.4 per cent in UF sample; 30.0 per cent in the ESF sample); 'three or four times a week' (31.5 per cent in the UF sample; 34.0 per cent in the ESF sample) 'every day' (41.1 per cent in the UF sample; 36.0 per cent in the ESF sample). For the ESF analysis, the categories 'at least once a month' and 'at least once a week' were aggregated in the category 'one or two times a week or less frequently'.
8 All results of non-parametric correlations presented in this chapter have been previously checked with results obtained through cross-tabulations and other descriptive techniques. The significance levels of coefficients presented through-out the paper are reported as follows: ** means significance at the 0.01 level; * means significance at 0.05 level. Where a dichotomous variable was used, we carried out a Chi Square Test (where the variable was crossed with another dichotomous variable) and a Mann-Whitney U Test (where the variable was crossed with an ordinal variable).
9 For the ESF sample, the indicators aggregated in the additive index were dichotomous variables concerning the following forms of action: convincing someone to vote for a party, signing a petition/referendum, leafleting, striking, participating in a sit-in, boycotting, occupying abandoned buildings, committing violence against property. For the UF sample, the index was generated by the aggregation of the following indicators of political participation: striking, supporting an electoral campaign, participating in a peaceful demonstration, participating in a disruptive demonstration, occupying abandoned houses, occupying abandoned buildings.

10 For both samples, the indicators aggregated in the additive index were dichotomous variables concerning the following organisations: political party, trade union, voluntary group (charity), NGO, religious group, student group, social centre. In the UF research the index also included leisure associations. In the ESF research the index also included women's association, environmental association and pro-immigrants association.

11 For the ESF sample, the additive index included four indicators: visiting a website of any source of 'alternative information', signing online petitions or participating in campaigns through email and/or mailing-lists, expressing political or social opinions in forums/mailing lists/chats, participating in a net-strike and/or in other forms of online radical protest. In the case of the UF sample the additive index included five indicators, of which two referred to the electoral campaign of 2001 (using the Internet to get information, forwarding emails containing political propaganda) and three referred to no specific event (receiving emails with political or social-minded contents, expressing political or social opinions in forums/mailing lists/chats, participating in 'awareness campaigns').

12 The results of a non-parametric test for two independent samples (Mann-Whitney U Test) are: UF (Z −1.663); ESF (Z −2.121*). Gender is distributed as follows: in the UF sample 63 per cent are female; in the ESF sample 48 per cent are female. Age is distributed as follows: in the UF sample 33 per cent are 25 years old or older, 41 per cent are between 22 and 24, and 26 per cent are 21 or younger. In the ESF sample 20 per cent are 25 years old or older, 40 per cent are between 22 and 24, and 40 per cent are 21 or younger.

13 The only difference is that females are less likely to participate in disruptive or unconventional and illegal actions such as occupying abandoned buildings and participating in disruptive demonstrations.

14 In both questionnaires an indicator of the political orientation of students was included. Originally, we used two different Likert scales: in the UF research we used a 5-point scale while in the ESF research we used a 7-point scale running from extreme left to extreme right. Unsurprisingly, due to the characteristics of the samples, we observed a concentration of students in the radical and moderate left positions on the scale. This concentration on the left is highest in the ESF sample, which mirrors the political orientation of the participants in the movement against neo-liberal globalisation. For the ESF sample the distribution across the political continuum is as follows: 27 per cent define themselves as radical leftist (1), 55 per cent as leftist (2), 15 per cent as centre-leftist (3), while only 3 per cent placed themselves on the centre-right of the political spectrum (4-7). In the UF sample the distribution is as follows: 39 per cent define themselves as leftist (1), 50 per cent as centre-leftist (2), 8 as centre (3), with only 3 per cent placing themselves on the centre-right (4-5).

15 We found political orientation useful to describe the characteristics of students. However, in the section that follows we decided not to use this to interpret political Internet use, because of its redundancy with indicators of political participation.

16 In Table 6.1 the indicators of political action (described in the paragraph 'Characteristics of the research') are aggregated in two different categories that refer to 'non-radical' and 'radical' forms of participation. For both samples, the indicators included in the additive index of radical actions were dichotomous variables comprising the following: occupying abandoned buildings (ESF and UF); participating in a disruptive demonstration and occupying abandoned houses (only UF); committing violence against property (only ESF). Other indicators cited in note 8 (i.e. those differing from those mentioned above) were used to generate the additive index of non-radical actions.

17 It is important to clarify that the highest rates of organisational participation in the ESF sample may be partly explained by the fact that in this study the question referred to present and past experiences, while in the UF sample the question referred only to present participation.

18 The category 'other civil society organisations' includes: environmental associations, student groups and social centres (in both studies) while the ESF research also includes women's and pro-immigrants' groups.

19 We checked this trend with the statistics drawn from the original version of the UF sample, which included 380 cases and in which the students represented the entire political spectrum. We found that political orientation was negatively correlated with political action (-0.543**). In particular, we found that in moving to the extreme right of the political spectrum, participation in peaceful demonstrations (-0.351**) and strikes (-0.352**) decreased, followed by 'contributing to electoral campaigns' (-0.234**) and 'being active in a political party' (-0.188**).

20 The result of the Mann-Whitney U Test between the indicator of participation in a demonstration on globalization issues and the political use of the Internet index is Z -2.284*.

21 The question was 'How much do you trust the mass media?'.

22 The question was 'Have you ever discussed social or political issues on the Internet through posting or sending messages in forums, mailing-lists or chat rooms?'.

23 The low number of cases in the UF sample (N = 4) did not allow for a specific analysis.

24 In the UF survey we asked students if they had ever contributed to the diffusion of online awareness campaigns and, if yes, through which means they did it. 50 per cent of students had and the most selected tools were 'forwarding messages to others' (49 per cent) and 'signing a petition' (27 per cent).

7 Australian young people's participatory practices and Internet use

Ariadne Vromen

The Internet is often portrayed as a democratising agent able to facilitate participatory practices. Alternatively, the advent of the Internet is also seen as a contributor to a new class divide; a digital divide between those who access and utilise technology and information, and those who do not, or cannot. It is often assumed that young people are the big winners in the Internet revolution. This chapter discusses these ideas in the Australian context through a focus on three areas: demographic differences and Internet use; the relationship between political participation, broadly defined, and Internet use; and case studies of organisations that facilitate young people's Internet based participation.

Based on original survey data, this chapter examines the relationship between Internet use and political participation among Australian young people. Based on original survey data it demonstrates that there clearly exists a 'digital divide' delineated on demographic characteristics of geography, education level, income level and occupational classification. While the Internet has far from replaced traditional information sources of television and newspapers, it does, however, facilitate participation undertaken by already politically engaged young people. The Internet has fundamental importance in facilitating information sharing and organising for young people involved in activist and community groups. The chapter also introduces two brief case studies of non-government, youth-oriented organisations with participatory Internet sites to further explore the potential of Internet enhancement of young people's autonomous political spaces.

Literature review

Evaluating debates on whether the Internet facilitates political engagement, Pippa Norris (2001: 96–8) differentiates between 'cyber-optimists' and 'cyber-sceptics'. Cyber-optimists believe that the unlimited information available through the Internet will foster an increase in political knowledge, that people will express their views freely on email, lists and in chat rooms, and will subsequently become more active in community politics. This view encapsulates the mobilisation thesis, which sees that the Internet has the capacity to engage those currently on the periphery of the existing political systems – such as young people, those living in non-urban communities, or those disillusioned with the mainstream political system (ibid. 2001: 218). Cyber sceptics, in contrast, see that the Internet will be used politically for reinforcement by those citizens already active and knowledgeable about political and community affairs. Therefore, those with this view suggest that the Internet will not change existing levels of participation, and could even widen the gap between the engaged and those who are politically indifferent (ibid.: 218, 98).

Others have argued that the Internet provides new ways of participating in political processes, and thus merits distinctive analysis. For example, the rapid uptake of mobile phones, digital television and the Internet have all occurred in the last decade and Stanyer argues that this has created opportunities for an increase in individualised political expression and participation (Stanyer, 2005: 21). These individualised forms of participation include traditional modes such as voting, writing letters to MPs, donating money and non-traditional modes that are facilitated by new technology, including petition signing, boycotts, blogging, chat rooms, email chain letters and SMS (for example, to media and politicians). Non-traditional modes of individualised participation are often quicker, require little time commitment and are often convenient for expressing a political viewpoint (Stanyer, 2005: 22; Vromen and Gelber, 2005: 301–5). However, this research has not yet been utilised to explain how the Internet facilitates or underpins collective action, and/or political deliberation in general.

The ABS Report *Australia Online* (Lloyd and Bill, 2004) presents an overview of the home-based computer and Internet use of Australians utilising 2001 census data. Overall it finds that there are a range of socio-economic and demographic factors that account for differences in the rates of technology use. The main characteristics of those who use the Internet regularly are:

- those with high weekly family incomes;
- those with high level of education; or still in school and study;
- families with dependent children;
- the employed, and in white collar jobs, especially professional occupations;
- younger people, especially those under 25;
- those living in cities rather than regional or rural Australia;
- people exposed to computer and Internet use in the workplace.

The research found that young Australians under the age of 25 are by far the greatest users of the Internet. However, correlations between the socio-economic factors showed that technology (especially Internet) use and income were more strongly associated than technology use and age (Lloyd and Bill, 2004: 23, 85). This starts to suggest that Australian young people, especially when they are no longer studying, cannot all be categorised as active Internet users. Understanding and predicting general Internet usage is more likely to rely on the complex interaction between the demographic characteristics listed above, especially those that indicate high socioeconomic status.

This chapter focuses especially on the relationships between Internet use and political participation broadly defined. In the recent literature I found four main ways of analysing the relationship between Internet use and young people's political participation and engagement. First, research often focuses on the Internet as an alternative and readily engaging service provider, principally for disadvantaged or at risk young people (for example, Lock *et al.*, 2002). Thus, targeted Internet services that provide anonymity, speed of response and privacy are represented as appealing to young people who are comfortable with utilising the technology. This focus on alternate modes of providing services is clearly generationally specific although there is minimal analysis of how Internet usage in general is concentrated among the affluent and highly educated who may have less immediate need for targeted services.

There is a second, broader discussion of the potential for activism facilitated by the Internet. The anti-globalisation movement has been noted for the way it utilises Internet-based media and information delivery through email used for protest organisation; and Indymedia which often uses live action footage relayed through websites. Activist organisations more broadly, such as Greenpeace or Oxfam Community Aid Abroad, have been adept at using the Internet to provide information and foster the participation and involvement of individuals (see Barr, 2002: 252; Scalmer, 2002; Iveson and Scalmer, 2000). Graham Meikle (2002) believes that the Internet has provided a new tool for those who intend to create social and political change, but that this tool works together with existing media forms. For example, political activists use and create Internet based alternatives for news and political commentary sources, such as Indymedia, but they also need to promote their issues by receiving coverage in more widely accessed media such as television and metropolitan newspapers.

Others have commented on how the alternative media space provided by the Internet facilitates alternative political agendas (Evans 2004). However, Evans hastens to add that virtual communities are not necessarily more democratic or inclusive than physical communities, and that most people still find inclusion through traditional community forms in physical spaces (Evans, 2004).

The third area of discussion takes up this idea of the Internet's provision of alternative political outlets and focuses on how the Internet makes it possible for young people to create new and distinctive political spaces. Bessant (2000: 115) cites as examples Internet-based discussion of racism and subsequent actions organised to protest against Pauline Hanson (who started the far right One Nation political party) in 1998. She argues that this example: 'illustrates how the net can help empower young people and how such technology can shape and influence the content of political practice for some young people.' Similarly, Anita Harris (2001) describes alternative spaces and forums for political expression created by young women ranging from underground magazines to alternative music to 'gURL' web pages (see also Cross, 1996 on geekgirl). It is the Internet that facilitates unregulated communication between young women, and gives them the opportunity to have political exchanges that are not appropriated, misunderstood or even seen by those not invited in.

In this view the Internet offers potential for a more personal and private politics. That is, young people are able to participate in discussion and information sharing without being evaluated by either their peers or others in civil society. It is this construction of the Internet as providing an autonomous and alternative forum for politics that is both difficult to measure and/or ignored in studies of participation. It is important that studies of young people's utilisation of the Internet now incorporate this qualitative focus on the new spaces that are created and used by young people. It is only then that we will be able to understand whether the use of the Internet can progress from fostering individualised participation into more collectively-oriented participation with the capacity to foster deliberation.

The fourth area of research and analysis is a focus on the individual level relationship between Internet use and social capital. To some extent this discussion lays the groundwork for an examination of whether there is a relationship between Internet use and group-based participation. Social capital is generally depicted as a conceptual approach to measuring both connections within communities and individual levels of civic engagement (see Winter, 2000). As social capital looks at how people engage and connect within geographic and identity based communities it is a useful contributor to the broad-based definition of political participation. In the Australian policy-making context a recent Productivity Commission (2003: 55) report suggested that governments could facilitate social capital in communities by funding Internet and telecommunications services, thus bridging disadvantage and the 'digital divide'. Research undertaken in North America (Quan-Haase and Wellman, 2002: 3) has suggested that there are three different approaches to conceptualising the effects the Internet has on social capital accumulation:

1   The Internet transforms social capital. In that the Internet provides the capacity for communication with distant communities of shared interest; and thus the Internet creates *new* communities.
2   The Internet diminishes social capital, in that the Internet chiefly entertains and draws people away from family and friends, and thus the Internet leads to *less* community.
3   The Internet supplements social capital. The Internet is a part of people's everyday lives and another means of communication, facilitating existing relationships and patterns of civic engagement and community building.

The existing research tends to confirm the third approach to the Internet social capital accumulation relationship. That is, the Internet has not radically transformed or mobilised civic engagement despite that active community groups use the Internet extensively (Quan-Haase *et al.*, 2002: 9; Shah *et al.*, 2001: 155–6).

Shah *et al.*'s (2001: 149, 155) quantitative study of the relationship between individual Internet use, civic engagement and generations found that there was a significant but weak relationship between Internet use and civic engagement. This relationship was strongest amongst adults below the age of 34. This study was important because it examined Internet use in terms of both overall usage and what it was used for. However, the study's limitations are in the operationalisation of civic engagement, which relied on only three indicators of: 'did volunteer work', 'worked on a community project' and 'went to a club meeting' (2001: 146). Arguably these three indicators do not extend to broader instances of political participation nor do they provide the opportunity to examine political and community involvements that may be specific to young people (for a more extensive critique of narrow indicators of participation and civic engagement see Vromen, 2003; Ester and Vinken, 2003 and the discussion in the Method section below).

This chapter extends on these different types of political uses of the Internet that were identified in the existing literature. This included individualistic uses for formal and less formal political engagement, collectively oriented uses for both social capital oriented civic engagement, as well as activist politics. The chapter evaluates these different uses in the Australian context by, first, focusing on broad quantitative patterns of how young people use the Internet and the relationship with their participatory practices. This analysis evaluates whether the Internet is used to reinforce existing participation or mobilise new groups of young people to participation. We then shift to case study-oriented research of two non-government organisations that utilise the Internet to foster young people's engagement and participation: a service-oriented youth site and a discussion-based culturally-oriented youth site. These case studies suggest the importance of focusing on the construction of particular political spaces not universalising patterns of individual behaviour alone.

Method

We draw on a survey of a broadly representative sample of 287 18- to 34-year-old Australians conducted via telephone by Newspoll Market Research in 2001. Respondents were selected by the application of a stratified random sample process that included: a quota set for each Australian capital city and non-capital city areas, within each of these areas a quota was set for each telephone area code; random selection of household telephone numbers that were drawn from current telephone listings for each area code; and random selection of an individual in each household by screening questions requesting the resident individual who last had a birthday. I designed the survey in consultation with the polling company.

This data-set has both strengths and limitations. It is a new data-set that focuses on political participation, and in a more extensive way than existing explorations of young people's political practices. However, I acknowledge that the generalisability of the results are limited by the small sample size, and there may be some reservations about the broad age range of young people surveyed. I nonetheless consider that it is important to look at a broader age group of young people to understand the complex relationship between generational change, participation and technology. Other studies have broadened the usual policy-making and institutionalised notions of youth, as age 15 to 25 (see Wyn and White, 1997: 1), to extend to the late twenties (see Hillman and Marks, 2002; Dwyer *et al.*, 1998). I extended the age group being studied to 34 to be able to measure social and economic change experienced by a generation of Australian young people and in acknowledgement that age-based trajectories, or markers, in both the public and private sphere are not as predictable as they once were (for example, Shah *et al.*, 2001; White and Wyn, 2004). In Australia several life course markers no longer occur within the usual demarcations of the 'youth' into 'adult' age group: these include life-course events such as leaving the parental home, becoming financially independent, entering a partnership, having children or buying a house (see Hillman and Marks, 2002).

I developed the questionnaire topics so as to account for a broad range of participatory activities. This included 19 activities such as the boycotting of products, and a range of community and activist group involvements (see Table 7.1); as well as issues that young people discuss, and the perceived constraints on time they had available for participation, but these are not analysed here. The questionnaire did not ask individuals to estimate the amount of time they spent participating in any of the participatory activities or groups. This was judged as too complicated and temporally dependent for a single highly structured interview. This kind of information can only be reliably collected through time use diaries, preferably in a longitudinal panel study. I was also more interested in elaborating on the *range* of, and relationships between, participatory activities undertaken by individuals, rather than trying to calculate the time spent on different participatory acts.

I have argued elsewhere that traditional indicators of participation that rely on labelling some types of participation as conventional and other types of participation as unconventional tends to both belittle and diminish our capacity to understand young people's participation. That is, conventional political behaviour research establishes a hierarchy of participation that more often than not measures young people's lack of interest in formal politics as an indicator of their political apathy. By including a broad range of individualised, community and activist involvements in my measurements

Table 7.1 Forms of political participation

Activist (7 items)	
Human rights organisation	Environmental organisation
Women's organisation	Heritage/conservation organisation
Attended rally or march	Boycotted products
Other activist organisation	
Communitarian (6 items)	
Church group	Youth club
Volunteered time	School/university group
Contacted MP	Ethnicity group
Party (5 items)	
Campaign work	Party member
Union member	Contacted MP
Sporting/recreation group	
Individualistic (4 items)	
Volunteered time	Made donations
Boycotted products	Sporting/recreation group

of young people's participation it has been possible to more accurately gauge young people's extensive level of engagement with broad-based political issues and processes (Vromen, 2003).

In constructing my questionnaire I did make a choice in favour of quantitative, generalisable breadth, over qualitative depth of analysis, so as to be able to locate patterns apparent in the population (see Sanders, 2002; May, 2001: 89). However, a complex and well-rounded understanding of participation cannot be obtained without *also* looking at the qualitative and contextual dimensions to participatory practice (see Bryman, 1998). Which is why I have adopted Dunleavy's (1996) call for methodological pluralism by also focusing on particular Internet usage through the case studies of youth-led Internet sites of two organisations: Vibewire Youth Services and Inspire Foundation. I have also addressed Dunleavy's suggestion that disaggregation is needed in behavioural research, by looking for divergent patterns within the age group being studied rather than stressing homogenous patterns of participation. In an earlier paper I explored the 19 acts of participation in detail (Vromen, 2003), and undertook factor analysis that led to identification of four types of participation: communitarian, activist, individualistic and party-oriented. In this chapter I focus on the relationship between use of the Internet and acts of political participation.

Sourcing information and Internet use

This section details the findings on young people's use of the Internet in general and how it is related to their participatory practices in particular.

The results here reinforce common assumptions about media usage in that nearly all young people generally use television to find out about the world (94 per cent), and it is the most commonly used main source of information (47 per cent). However, other mass media forms, that is newspapers (84 per cent, most common: 25 per cent) and radio (74 per cent, most common: 14 per cent), continue to also be important sources of information about news and current affairs. Young Australians are clearly differentiated into those who are actively online and those who are not, as only 45 per cent of the sample use the Internet generally as a source of information, and only 6 per cent say the Internet is their main source of information.

In examining young people's general Internet use 34 per cent use the Internet every day, and 66 per cent use at least email regularly, that is at least once a week. They mainly use the Internet for work and study, or for communicating with friends and family. A smaller proportion use it for finding out about entertainment, sport, news and current affairs and community events. A very small group (8 per cent) agree that they use the Internet for sharing information about community or political issues. Nineteen per cent of the sample never use the Internet. The primary differentiating demographic characteristics of the non-Internet users are that they tend to be less educated, have a main income earner working in blue-collar work and to be in a household that earns less money than the sample's average.

Table 7.2 Internet usage

	Email (%)	Internet (exc. email) (%)
Every day	46	34
1–3 times a week	20	29
Less often, or never	34	37

Table 7.3 Reasons for Internet use

Use	Percentage
For work or study reasons	78
Keep in touch with family and friends	77
To find out about:	
Entertainment/sporting events	47
News and current affairs	40
Community events	17
Share information about community or political issues	8
Other	22

Note: The 'other' category included mentions of items such as: Internet banking and shopping, holiday information and bookings, downloading and playing games and music, and general entertainment.

Email and Internet usage were examined to see if they differed along nine demographic variables. There was no difference among the three age groups (18–24, 25–29, 30–34), which means that while work and study are important reasons for using the Internet it is not necessarily the youngest group, 18- to 24-year-olds, who are the most Internet active. Frequency of use for both email and Internet did differ significantly along the predictable class-oriented demographics of location, education level, income level and occupational classification. City dwellers were more likely than their regional rural counterparts to use both email and the Internet everyday. A minority of those who had not completed secondary school (23 per cent) compared to majority of those with secondary school (51 per cent) or post-secondary school qualifications (56 per cent) used email everyday; the pattern was similar for frequency of Internet usage. Those in the highest income bracket were much more likely to use email everyday (63 per cent) and only 22 per cent of those in the lowest income bracket used the Internet every day. The sample also divides around white- and blue-collar work, with 52 per cent of blue-collar workers using email and the Internet less often than once a week. The existence of these relationships demonstrates that there clearly is a 'digital divide' among younger Australians, in terms of the frequency of their usage of both email and the Internet. While there was no difference between men and women for the frequency of their email use, a difference does appear when it comes to Internet use in that men (41 per cent) are more likely than women (26 per cent) to use the Internet everyday. Reasons for Internet use are explored below, but suffice to say that gender difference does not reappear along any of these indicators. One of the more interesting findings is that people from a non-English speaking background (NESB) use the Internet more frequently than people from an English speaking background, with only 13 per cent of NESB individuals saying that they use the Internet less than once a week. This suggests that the Internet has broadened opportunities for NESB individuals in terms of the resources that they can access in their language of origin.

The reasons for people using the Internet were examined by the demographic variables. The higher level of education gained, the more likely individuals will use the Internet for work and study: 85 per cent of those with a post-secondary school qualification use the Internet for work or study, compared to 62 per cent of those who have not finished school. This probably relates to the nature of work and study for those with more education, in that their work may be professionalised, more dependent on information technology and thus reinforces the notion of the 'digital divide'. No other demographic indicators differentiate the group who use the Internet for work and study.

People from a non-English speaking background differ from those of an English speaking background when it come to two particular uses of the Internet. NESB Australians are much more likely to use the Internet to find about news and current affairs than their ESB counterparts (67 per cent compared to 36 per cent). They are also somewhat more likely to us the Internet to find out about community events (17 per cent to 7 per cent). This suggests that people from a non-English speaking background are turning to the Internet to fulfil an information need that is not being fully met by mainstream media. It could be assumed that this is information on news and community events that is written in the other language spoken at home. Dividing the sample into different demographic groups does not help us to understand inclination toward any other uses of the Internet. That is, men and women, different income groups, different work status, parent and non-parents, city and rural residents, and different age groups all use the Internet for more or less the same reasons. Overall these results imply that there is a digital divide among Australian young people in terms of frequency of email and Internet use, but there are very few demographic differences in terms of what the Internet is actually being used for. In the following section I ascertain whether there is a relationship between acts of participation and Internet usage.

Participation and Internet use

In this research I used 19 different participatory acts that ranged from individualised activities aimed at institutionalised actors, such as government, to protest-based activities, to collective group involvements. The 19 acts of participation were analysed to determine whether certain acts statistically factored together, that is whether individuals were predisposed to engage in a certain range of participatory acts. Four factors were identified and I labelled them as: activist; communitarian; party and individualistic (listed in Table 7.1). Most people have engaged in the individualistic activities, such as volunteering time or making a donation. The collective, group-based activities included in both the communitarian and activist factors appeal to distinctive, but separate, groups within this generation of young people. The party-based factor that includes party membership had limited, and diminishing, appeal to young people (Vromen, 2003; also see McAllister, 1997: 247).

Analysis was undertaken to see if there were relationships between both the amount of time people used the Internet and what they used it for, with the acts of political participation. Overall, there was little significant relationship between everyday use of the Internet (and email) and individual acts of participation. Thus a prior involvement in a single participatory activity does not lead to, nor is it influenced by, frequent email and Internet use.

A significant relationship was found between the number of participatory acts that a person engages in and the frequency of their email and Internet use. Therefore, individuals who use both email and the Internet every day were significantly more involved in a range of acts of participation. This suggests that as people are more open to a range of participatory acts they may use email and the Internet both to communicate more and access further information. These individuals are subsequently predisposed to participation and information. However, this can also potentially be attributed to the strong relationship of both education level and occupational status with both Internet use and participation.

I also examined the relationship between the four participatory factors (activist, communitarian, party and individualist) and email and Internet use. There are no significant relationships between frequency of email use and the participatory factors. Furthermore, Internet usage did not relate to either the party or individualist participatory factors. However, where the results became interesting is in the statistical relationships between Internet usage and the two collective group-based factors: the activist and communitarian types. Individuals who use the Internet every day and weekly both have a significantly higher average on both group-based participatory factors than do those who use the Internet rarely. This suggests a level of interdependence between use of the Internet as an information source and as a tool for political engagement. It may also suggest that those predisposed to activist and community-based participation utilise the Internet as a source of information alternative to the mainstream media that does not regularly cover issues of interest or relevance to those involved in community-based or activist pursuits.

Reasons for using both the Internet and email were also examined for any relationship with the participatory factors. All four types of participation were found to have a significant relationship with both individuals' use of the Internet for finding out about community/political events and sharing information about these events. While individuals who use the Internet for these two reasons have a higher average on each of the four participatory factors, it is difficult to understand which actions come first. That is, do people who participate more use the Internet more as a normal course to sustain their participation *or* are people who use the Internet for a broader range of reasons more likely to become politically active in non-Internet based participation? This is the trade-off described by Pippa Norris (2001) between the reinforcement and mobilisation effects that the Internet has on participation.

I suspect that young people use the Internet to facilitate existing forms of participation because there is also a significantly higher average on all four participatory factors for those who use the Internet for work and study. Thus Internet use in people's everyday lives is also related to higher levels of participation in general. For example, individuals who use the Internet to either keep in touch with family and friends or for work and study reasons have a higher average on the activist factor than those who do not use the Internet for those reasons, suggesting that activists are increasingly Internet savvy or even Internet dependent, and their participation moulds to those predispositions.

Table 7.4 Participatory factors' relationship with reasons for Internet use

		Average for those who use the Internet for this reason	Average for those who do not use the Internet for this reason	Level of significance
Activist	Work/study	1.7	1.1	**
	Keep in touch	1.7	1.1	**
	Finding out community info	2.1	1.4	*
	Sharing community info	2.9	1.4	*
Communitarian	Work/study	2.1	1.6	*
	Finding out community info	2.7	1.8	**
	Sharing community info	2.9	1.8	**
Party	Work/study	1.5	1.2	*
	Finding out entertainment	1.6	1.3	*
	Sharing community info	2.1	1.4	*
Individualist	Work/study	3	2.7	*
	Finding out community info	3.3	2.8	*
	Sharing community info	3.7	2.8	**
Total acts	Work/study	6.1	4.7	**
	Keep in touch	5.9	4.9	*
	Finding out entertainment	6.1	5.2	*
	Finding out community info	7	5.3	**
	Sharing community info	8.6	5.3	**

About one third of the 19 individual participatory acts have a significant relationship with the two Internet uses of either finding or sharing information on community and political affairs. The associations here are relatively weak, but it is clear that activist acts such as attending a rally and boycotting are facilitated by political exchanges through the Internet. Furthermore, a series of group-based formations, both community and activist oriented are associated with use of the Internet for these community/politically oriented reasons. However, these findings can also be traced back to education levels, as the highly educated are more likely to be participatory, more likely to use the Internet and much more likely to have been involved with a group at either school or university.

Interestingly, using the Internet to access information on news and current affairs is not significantly related to high levels of participation, either overall or on the four participatory factors. All those who look for news on the Internet are equally participatory. That is, while seeking out news and current affairs is an important reason for using the Internet it does not delineate people along the participatory factors. This result, added to the result that there is no relationship between Internet use and discussion

Table 7.5 Individual acts of participation with Internet use: finding out and sharing information on community/political events

Use of the Internet	Participatory act (% of sample)	% of participants who have used Internet for community/political reasons	Strength of association and significance level
Finding out information community events			
	School/university Group (37)	22	0.175*
	Rally (19)	26	0.167*
	Boycott (57)	18	0.128*
	Contact MP (24)	21	0.123*
	Church group (27)	21	0.12*
	Youth club (25)	21	0.115*
Sharing information on community events			
	Rally (19)	17	0.195**
	Boycott (57)	10	0.176*
	School/university group (37)	12	0.176*
	Women's group (9)	19	0.173*
	Sporting group (70)	9	0.144*
	Environment group (22)	13	0.127*
	Volunteered (67)	9	0.126*

of topical community and political issues, reinforces that participation and Internet use are related when the Internet reinforces existing 'real world' participation. Overall, the Internet is not used by the general population of young people as an alternative forum for community and political discussion.

This does not mean, conversely, that the Internet is not providing important political space for active young people. While I have demonstrated here that the Internet is not providing a radical change for young people in general by facilitating new participation I still suspect that it has made fundamental changes to the ways of participating for particular activist and community-oriented young people. That is, the Internet has now become indispensable for a variety of reasons such as, information distribution, sharing news and information, event organisation, keeping in contact, and for facilitating debate within both offline and Internet based communities. As I suggested at the beginning of this chapter, little research has explored how young people create Internet spaces that are autonomous and aid in deliberation. In the next section I make preliminary observations about two Internet sites to provoke further analysis of how Australian young people are already using the Internet in both political and deliberative ways.

Youth-led Internet spaces

In policy discussion of e-democracy or e-governance there has been limited discussion of the implementation of Internet based processes that actively include young people. Moreover, in this discussion a limited notion of Internet based participation is followed, one that tends to focus on government directed information delivery and consultation with individuals rather than active processes of citizen ownership and collective forms of participation (see, for example, the report of the recent Victorian Government's inquiry into Electronic Democracy http://www.parliament. vic.gov.au/sarc/E-Democracy/Final_Report). There are some Australian-based examples of government-led Internet initiatives that are targeted at young people (for example, see the Queensland government's Generate and the federal government's The Source http://www.thesource.gov.au/) but these tend to be similarly limited in their participatory potential. Existing survey research on the Australian third sector's general use of Internet sites to facilitate participation shows that very few organisations (less than 20 per cent) provide opportunities for collective oriented deliberation through discussion forums or actions. Most do, however, facilitate individualised participation such as donations, information access and merchandising purchases (Barraket, 2005: 26–7).

The United Kingdom is more advanced than Australia in the policy discussion and policy implementation of Internet-based facilitation of young people's political engagement. However, one major criticism of existing government and community sector led strategies in the UK is the lack of ownership and control young people have of producing and designing Internet content aimed at facilitating youth participation (Howland, 2002: 23).

Following my earlier definitions of a broad based approach to measuring and evaluating political participation I selected two youth oriented websites that facilitate young people's active engagement with society more broadly but are not necessarily always focused on formal politics. Through looking at these types of sites it is possible to better evaluate the extent of young people's agency in deliberating on issues that are directly important in their everyday lives. These brief case studies of two Australian non-government, non-profit organisations that provide youth targeted websites – Inspire Foundation and Vibewire Youth Services – show that both organisations actively facilitate the involvement of young people in website content and general direction of the organisations sponsoring the websites.

Inspire Foundation was formed in 1996 in response to Australia's unacceptably high rates of youth suicide and attempted suicide, and the intention of Inspire Foundation is to create opportunities for young people to help themselves and help others. The organisation has pioneered the use of the Internet and its associated technologies in creating and delivering new forms of social services for young people. Inspire argue that their services are effective because the Internet is the medium of young people, and can be used anonymously 24 hours a day. Inspire provides Reach Out! a service-oriented site that provides information and advice on general issues of young people's mental health. It is an award winning site and has a high level of interactivity. Inspire has recently established ActNow a new site that will facilitate young people's political and community engagement.

Vibewire Youth Services was established in 2001 to provide a primarily Internet-based youth media space. Its main plank Vibewire.net went live in April 2002 as a portal for youth culture and political expression. It provides a range of different sections where articles are posted and forums are conducted. Topics covered include: politics, policy and public issues; and cultural commentary on the areas of art, music, poetry, literature, film and theatre. In 2004 and 2005 Vibewire ran Sanctuary in partnership with Auburn Migrant Resource centre; this programme focused on the idea of multiculturalism and was aimed at giving young people from non-English speaking backgrounds the chance to publish creative work challenging the views of society on migrants and refugees. In 2004 Vibewire was also funded by the Foundation for Young Australians to run electionTracker whereby four young people wrote articles on the 2004 federal election campaign. These online journalists wrote daily entries on the website from the campaign trails of either Prime Minister John Howard or Leader of the Opposition Mark Latham. Opinion pieces by the four electionTrackers were also reprinted in mainstream print media and there were several radio and television stories on the project.

Both organisations have undertaken survey based work to gain an overview of the users of their websites. Inspire commissioned Whetstone at The Leading Edge to undertake a short survey on their site in late 2002/early 2003. This self-selecting survey of nearly 1,000 users found that 80 per cent were female and the average age was 18. Most users were metropolitan based, and many of those were in Sydney. Site users were most likely to access the site because 'they were going through a hard time' and online links and promotions on youth radio station JJJ were the main ways of hearing about the Reach Out! site (Inspire Foundation, 2003).

In 2004 Vibewire distributed a survey on young people's media use primarily through their website but also through several off-line youth and media oriented forums. Similar to Inspire's findings, most of the 700 respondents were female (70 per cent) and metropolitan based (81 per cent); most respondents were between 20 and 25 years of age, and nearly 70 per cent were either fulltime or part time students. Evidenced by findings on participatory behaviour this sample was clearly a highly educated and politicised sample of young people who are not representative of young Australians in general. In terms of Internet based participation two thirds of the respondents had participated in an online forum, 40 per cent had written an article for a website and one third had run their own website (Vibewire, 2005).

Beyond both appealing disproportionately to women the two sites seem to have different audiences, thus representing their different missions. Vibewire seems to be providing an outlet for young people who are highly educated and engaged with media, and social and political debates in general. These young people are demographically similar to both the activist and communitarian participatory types I found in my survey-based research. It remains to be seen whether Vibewire is mobilising young people who were not previously politically engaged, but they are definitely providing a targeted outlet for political expression, through pulse, electionTracker and (federal) budgetTracker, of a kind that was not previously available. Inspire relies on active offline participation of young people to maintain an appropriate service for young people on broad issues of their mental health. It recently launched ActNow, which is deliberately focused on facilitating young people's civic and political engagement. The organisation sees that the Internet is the appropriate medium to foster both online and offline communities, with this new service they also are trying to demonstrate how active participation underpins the successful delivery of *all* their services for young people.

In terms of participation, Vibewire is more clearly run by and for young people – it has limited paid staff opportunities but all the volunteer young people administering the organisation, running the site and writing content must be under 30. Inspire is a much larger organisation in terms of funding and paid staff, and while not all the staff are young people most are: nine of its 19 staff are under 30, with another seven aged between 31 and 35. This suggests that working every day in youth services and in Internet-based services is attractive to young people. Inspire endeavours to maintain its legitimacy with young people more broadly through its two volunteer programmes: Reach Out! Youth Advisory Board and the subsequent Youth Ambassadors programme. Reach Out Youth Advisory Board members are primarily advisers to the website service – they are consulted on content, marketing and campaign ideas. There are three boards of approximately 15 young people each year, to make sure input to the service stays fresh and relevant. The approximately 130 youth ambassadors (most are 'graduates' of the advisory board) are active partners in the organisation's work and are more akin to volunteer staff members. They have a mandate to work with Reach Out! staff which includes writing content or conducting interviews for the site, sitting on staff interview committees and appearing in advertising campaigns. They also develop campaigns on mental health and Reach Out! within their broader offline communities and this is assisted by an annual skills workshop that Inspire runs in major capital cities.

Conclusions: democratising potential of Internet-based political practice

This research confirms the idea that there is an Australian digital divide between young people who are well educated, resourced and use the Internet, and those who do not have ready access to Internet technology and are not as socioeconomically advantaged. Furthermore, the relationship between participation and Internet usage seems to be one of reinforcement of existing political practices and persuasion, rather than of mobilisation of new political actors. The research does provide new quantitative evidence that the Internet facilitates information distribution and sharing for those involved in both activist and communitarian group based participation. The case studies of two non-government organisations that use the Internet to facilitate participation demonstrate the importance of youth-led political spaces for political engagement.

However, there is still much to learn about the way that young people use the Internet, and the potential relationships with political and community engagement. This research primarily looked at one facet of the Internet-political participation relationship through the focus on aggregated, individual specific data. There is a broader need for more in-depth qualitative or case study research on participation and Internet use. This research could start from several analytical points. First, a focus on individual attitudes towards politics and Internet use, especially in seeking to understand the motivations for those already highly engaged with the Internet in a political way. This could include interview research with those who construct Reach Out!, Act Now and vibewire.net and also the more private subjects of Anita Harris's (2001) research on young feminists' webzines.

Second, research could be commenced from political acts and organisations that are known to be attracting young people, such as environmental and human rights groups, protest and boycotting, to more comprehensively examine the relationship between the Internet and real-world participation. That is, asking these young people how they integrate the Internet with their active engagement and participation as well as treating it as a media-based socialisation source. These sorts of analyses could show whether the way the Internet is used by these politicised young people could assist in redeveloping governmental use of the Internet to encourage participation by a broader range of young people.

8 Rethinking online youth civic engagement

Reflections on web content analysis

Roman Gerodimos and Janelle Ward

Rethinking online youth civic engagement

Research on youth civic engagement is expanding, as scholars grow increasingly concerned about the state of participation in liberal democracies. The Internet is fast becoming an embedded part of teens' life world (Lenhart *et al.*, 2005) as well as a key domain of political interaction and communication. Understanding how young citizens communicate and participate – what their needs, motivations, gratifications and online preferences are – is vital in building tools of civic engagement that will facilitate their participation and, ultimately, empower them. At the same time it is necessary to evaluate what is on offer in terms of civic engagement spaces on the Internet.

Content analysis is a well-established method in many social science disciplines. Some define content analysis in a quantitative manner, as '... a research technique for the objective, systematic and quantitative description of the manifest content of communication' (Berelson, 1952: 18). Others see content analysis as encompassing a broader range of analytical possibilities, as 'any technique for making inferences by objectively and systematically identifying specified characteristics of a message' (Holsti, 1969: 14). Thus, content analysis can be conducted either in an interpretive fashion (i.e., a qualitative approach such as discourse analysis) or a more inferential one (i.e., a quantitative approach using statistical methods).

There has been a rapid rise in the number of studies using web content analysis (Weare and Lin 2000) although their scope is sometimes limited and usually quantitative, as in Gibson and Ward (2000). However, online researchers may be implementing inadequate analytical tools and, thus, risk misinterpretation. This shortfall stems from the fact that these tools are shaped in the offline world and correspond to more traditional or formal methods of participation. For example, some recent studies (Ward *et al.*, 2003; 2005) find that young people are not using the Internet to engage with traditional political activities (such as emailing their MPs) and are subsequently quite sceptical about the Internet's potential as a medium of political communication. Yet, such a conceptualisation of political participation may be overlooking a variety of other activities that young users engage with, and these activities could legitimately be considered as political. Indeed, such activities could themselves represent a redefinition of what we mean by 'politics'.

This chapter argues that both politics and the way we participate in public affairs are changing, and this change is partly due to the nature of new media and online communication. As a consequence, our analysis of online political content needs to adapt, especially when it comes to observing the younger generation.

In this chapter we first review the main parameters of evolution in political practice, linking it to youth culture and communication. Furthermore, we assess the challenges and opportunities created for content researchers with the rise of the Internet as a sphere of youth engagement. We also identify key differences between both online and offline content analysis and between traditional and emerging political practices. We complement our analysis with practical tips on how Internet researchers can improve their research strategies. We argue that the most effective research strategies are those that combine quantitative with qualitative elements; triangulate content analysis with either user or producer research that makes use of in-depth case studies (i.e., events, issues) or social networks/hyperlinked networks analyses as their sampling frameworks.

Allegedly, liberal democracies are facing a crisis of participation and legitimacy. This crisis is expressed through both political apathy and disengagement. The claim that citizens are disengaging from political processes is substantiated in trends such as deteriorating rates of voter turnout, a decline in social capital and voluntary associations, and a cultural gap between the world of political elites (for example, Washington DC, Westminster and Brussels) and the broader public. Gray and Caul (2000) attribute these patterns to the decline of group mobilisation in the second half of the twentieth century, while Rahn and Transue (1998) show that materialism and individualism among the younger generation is a key factor in the decline of social capital. The popularity of television shows such as *Big Brother* speaks to the masses' frustration with traditional political processes; recent research has shown striking and ever-expanding tensions between the two houses of Westminster and *Big Brother* (Coleman, 2003). These phenomena are said to be particularly evident with youth, not merely as an intracohort aberration, but as a mass, intergeneration shift that will continue to swell with each new generation (Putnam, 2000).

Yet, recent studies on youth attitudes towards participation and on their use of the Internet (Coleman and Rowe, 2005; Gerodimos, 2005; Lenhart *et al.*, 2004; Rainie and Horrigan, 2005; Smith *et al.*, 2005) demonstrate that young people are interested in, and are pursuing engagement with, public affairs, although outside of traditional institutions. In an extensive study of youth engagement websites in the United States, Montgomery *et al.*, (2004) describe this as a youth civic culture, particularly in relation to young people's civic and political activities online.

The four dimensions of change

Although many aspects of change are mentioned in terms of current youth civic disengagement, here we identify four dimensions especially relevant in an environment where both the perception of politics and the methods of online analysis are being re-evaluated. We include young people's response to the evolution of political content, space, time and reach.

The diffusion of the 'political'

As Internet use spreads throughout the population, young citizens find new and innovative ways to interact with others, absorb news, shape views and create their own content. Young people are often at the core of rising alternative forms of civic engagement and voice expression: culture-jamming and 'subvertising' (such as the AdBusters movement); flash-mobbing and impromptu protests; virtual networks spilling over to offline communities; the rise of citizen-reporters through blogging, vlogs and podcasts; online petitions, charity sites and other causes such as natural disaster aid. In the Pew Internet and American Life Project's study of online content creation, Lenhart *et al.*, (2004) find that young people are the most dynamic and creative group online; they largely comprise what is known as the 'power creators'. Moreover, Coleman and Rowe (2005: ii) find that 'it is not young people that are disconnected from formal politics, but political institutions that are disconnected from young people'. These young people, through practices such as sampling and remixing, are building their own culture online.

These findings concur with the conclusions of an extensive study by Ward *et al.* (2003: 665) on online participation in Britain. They found that 15- to 24-year-old users 'formed the biggest group of Internet-based participants, firmly displacing the middle-aged (45–54 years) who typically dominate in the offline world'. Moreover, they traced a 'very small, but distinct group of people who engaged only in online participation'.

This dispersion of voice expression and political participation via new media creates a fundamental challenge for the researcher. While sampling websites of formal political organizations is already complex, it is particularly difficult to build a sampling frame for web content analysis that takes into account virtual political expression and interaction. It essentially requires defining a boundary between what can and cannot be classified as political. This results in a complex predicament: the broader the definition of the political, the larger the potential pool of websites that can be sampled. Clearly, 'the question of which online activities merit the label of "participation" remains unresolved. What exactly must young people do online before society will judge them "politically active" or "engaged in civic participation"?' (Livingstone *et al.*, 2005: 289). For example, it may be reasonable to claim that the recent trend of charity wristbands was partly a conscious political act by young people who used this opportunity to express their concerns about global problems and, in doing so, to negotiate their identities as members of a collective. In that case, a corporate website might have been more relevant in terms of youth civic engagement than other non-corporate, perhaps governmental, websites.

However, even if the researcher is able to make a clear judgement about a website's relevant criteria so as to be considered both political and relevant to youth, it is very unlikely that they will be able to explicitly catalogue the entire population (or even a representative sample) of that particular type of site. In their study of sampling in web content analysis, Weare and Lin (2000: 273) argue: 'The sheer size and chaotic structure of the Internet . . . complicate[s] efforts to select representative samples of messages for analysis.'

One way to tackle this problem is to select a case study (one policy area or issue) and continue by conducting a qualitative, in-depth study of a small number of websites. Alternatively, another option would be to use a key site as a starting point and then, via hyperlink network analysis (Garrido and Halavais, 2003; Park, 2003), build a sampling frame that includes several degrees of separation to and from that site, resulting in a rigorous and systematic equivalent of snowball sampling. Farrall and Delli Carpini (2004) applied this method using an application called Issue Crawler on both the progressive left issue network and on the electronic voting issue network.

The collapse of space

The lack of clearly defined boundaries in the content of the online political sphere is not the only challenge facing web content researchers. Cyberspace is also defined by a total lack of physical or geographical boundaries which, as has been noted previously (Gerodimos, 2006), is a constituent feature of democracy. Specifically, how can democracy exist online when the 'demos' is unspecified? The reach of the old media is finite and, as a consequence, it is possible for social scientists to examine the media's political power, role and uses in reference to a particular national or local public sphere. Such rationale does not apply to the Internet, whose reach and use is global, taking into account the clearly significant limitations of access due to the digital divide. This is particularly true in the case of the so-called Internet generation, for whom the net is an embedded part of their everyday life.

Therefore, in the case of web content analysis it is virtually impossible to specify or delineate the audience and potential reach of the messages under analysis, while it may also be difficult to identify the creators of the messages. This is particularly true with synchronous and asynchronous spaces of virtual interaction (i.e., message boards and chat rooms) where the producers and receivers of messages cannot always be identified. Thus, a US site may be more influential to British youth than that of a UK-based organisation, as is the case with P2P file networks like Napster or Kazaa.

The collapse of space is facilitated by file sharing technology, as well as by the very culture and ideology of file sharers. While P2P can be merely seen as a leisure activity, some claim that it is actually a conscious, political act by the so-called 'online pirates'. Denegri-Knott (2004) argues that 'consumers committed to changing trading conditions engage in creative and innovative actions to traverse the field of actions established by an offline discourse'. The emerging (cyber) culture of resisting record companies is indicative of the changing power relations between consumers and established corporations.

Therefore, the distinction between national communication sources that would have been central in traditional content analyses becomes much less meaningful. For that reason, our sampling strategy needs to reflect the space – no longer exclusively local or national – where young citizens act politically and socially.

As in the previous case, focusing on a specific event or issue is a constructive way to narrow the focus of the research. A national issue or event, such as an election, a regional development or a local scandal may be easier to both sample online and to build a systematic framework of analysis, despite dissolving boundaries between local and global. There are numerous examples of so-called 'glocalized' (Wellman and Hampton, 1999) issues in dealing with environmental destruction and sustainability, immigration and asylum, and international trade, to name a few. Furthermore, we have recently witnessed a series of global events that have caused unprecedented public, mostly online mobilisation around the world, including 11 September, the Asian Tsunami and Hurricane Katrina in New Orleans.

Thus, web content researchers face the prospect of either restricting themselves to a limited set of methodologically manageable cases, or broadening to a more ambitious, topical agenda of global events that are often difficult to capture in a systematic way. The above-mentioned diffusion of wristbands in youth culture is typical of a global event that spread – primarily via the Internet – across countries and markets.

The collapse of time

As Internet scholars have previously noted (for example, see Castells, 1996), alongside the collapse of space online comes the collapse of time. Traditionally, content researchers have used key dates as a perimeter for their sampling frames. In performing a content analysis of media coverage of an election, scholars often examine relevant output at specific times during the election campaign (Jorgensen *et al.*, 1998; Scullion and Dermody,

2005; Smith and Smith, 2000). Alternatively, if a study focuses on an issue's 'natural history' in the media – thus utilising the concepts of framing or agenda-setting – they would collect material ranging from a few days to several months (McCombs, 1997; Simon and Xenos, 2000).

Yet, that type of sampling is becoming less useful due to the evolution of news production and consumption led by a variety of factors: the rise of the 24-hour news cycle; an evolution toward the 'permanent campaign'; and the appearance of 'accelerated pluralism', among other things. The rise of the 24-hour news cycle is a trend facilitated by the increase in cable, satellite and digital news networks like CNN or BBC World. Politics go on throughout the day and night, and relevant content is always available due to rolling coverage. Therefore, political communication is becoming both ubiquitous and continuous in practice. This is also reflected in the way Internet users access news, especially with young users who are becoming politically socialised within this new environment of choice, segmentation and information overload.

We have also witnessed a move towards the so-called permanent campaign (Ornstein and Mann, 2000). Election campaigns are now almost nominal: the real campaigning starts the day after the previous election. Furthermore, due to the increasing importance of image and presentation in political life (Franklin, 2004), political practice itself is more message-oriented with communication (along with decision making and implementation) being considered as one of the three key pillars of executive government. Scholars such as Street (1997) and van Zoonen (2004) argue that we are witnessing a fusion of politics with pop/youth culture.

In addition to these two shifts, the interactive and synchronous nature of the Internet further facilitates the multiplication of messages leading to what Bimber (1998) describes as accelerated pluralism. The rise of identity and issue politics and the proliferation of lobby groups and activist organisations accelerate the speed in which politics happens. Issues emerge, draw wide attention, are debated and then disappear from the limelight in shorter periods of time. Furthermore, online material is notoriously difficult to access over time. This represents a key difference between web content analysis and offline analysis. At present, we can still conduct content analyses of past newspaper articles and TV programmes. However, there is no reliable and accurate archive of online material, in that web pages can be modified hourly, defaced, or even permanently deleted. Researchers could, and have attempted to, thoroughly archive material, but such a process can lead to practical problems. Even if there were a reliable archive, the web is only a part of the Internet; there can be no reliable archive of all online activity in the last few decades. For example, while Google now offers an archive of most USENET newsgroups, threads and posts, authors and owners still reserve the right to remove publicly available material.

Digitisation fundamentally alters the nature of the material that content analysis has traditionally dealt with; it limits our options regarding the time of data collection. This is particularly evident when it comes to youth culture, which, in addition to its rapid change, often takes place outside well-established channels of communication. Lenhart *et al.* (2005: iii) find that 'instant messaging has become the digital communication backbone of teens' daily lives'.

Thus, it is much easier and more reliable to build a sampling frame and collect and analyse currently developing case or event data, rather than data on past events. Web content analysis on youth sites needs to be contemporary in the literal sense of the word; that is, the period of data collection needs to coincide with the duration of the event itself. Even hours after an issue has left the limelight of cyber culture, vital material could be lost or altered. That is not to say that one cannot conduct analyses of past material, but the most systematic and rigorous way to examine web content over time would need to be longitudinal analysis based on contemporaneous data collection. That said, one could question the importance of material that has very short shelf life online in studying youth civic engagement: web content that is visible for longer is potentially more likely to influence, or be used by, a greater number of young users. One example of this is interpersonal communication over email or instant messengers. Such communication is still an important variable in terms of youth awareness, discussion and even conflict, but it does not strictly fall under the heading of web content.

The 'pull' nature of the medium

The fourth element that challenges our traditional understandings and analyses of political messages is the segmentation of the material itself and the pull nature of the web, which encompasses all previously examined elements. Even if one were to construct a solid sampling frame for web content analysis that overcame the limitations and challenges set out above, there would still be the danger of analysing something that is irrelevant to what young citizens access or use (Livingstone *et al.*, 2005). In the national public sphere of the traditional broadcast media and in dominant political institutions, one could make some working assumptions (often based on actual ratings) about the receivers of a message, and that message's potential impact or reach.

Such assumptions are very difficult to construct in the case of the Internet, where equality dominates: Theoretically, at least, every voice and every byte has the same power as any other. Unless online content is 'picked up', that is, accessed and noticed by the user, there is no way to 'push' it to the audience. Some claim that young people are much more likely to use online collaborative sources than the established old media. Carroll (2004: 1) argues that '. . . newspaper readers are aging and dying off' while 'Generation Y's 16- to 24-year-olds . . . want to interact with the news, not merely to passively receive it'.

However, there is a danger in overstating the power of the Internet over that of the old media, or to be more accurate, the power of Internet-only organisations (for example, wikis or blogs) over those that were traditionally offline and then expanded on to the Internet. Big news organisations are still largely dominant as sources of news and entertainment as they are backed by multi-billion broadcast industries and perhaps more importantly, are part of the public's offline life.

One way to overcome this dilemma is by assessing the extent to which young citizens are using several functions and features of websites. A key strength of web content analysis is that without even leaving the site, the researcher can often analyse not just the political message itself but also the message's reception. Chat rooms, discussion and message boards may be considered as a vital element of youth websites that aim to create a sense of community and engagement. Therefore, measuring the quality and quantity of interaction present on such websites can help us evaluate the effectiveness of an online project's reach. Indeed, an analysis of youth parliament websites in the UK – such as the Scottish Youth Parliament and the Children and Young People's Assembly of Wales – showed that while these sites have built an extensive online structure with comprehensive coverage of political and youth issues, there is actually very limited interaction within the online community spaces (Gerodimos, 2005). Without obviously questioning the overall utility and reach of these websites, which is very difficult to establish without user research, at least one aspect of their agenda – that of online community and interaction – can be effectively assessed by web content analysis.

However, this is not only a problem of data collection or analysis: It is a sampling problem in the broader sense of analysing a corpus of websites that are relevant to people's everyday lives. This issue takes us back to the discussion surrounding the limits of the political. On the one hand, if the sites that young people actually use are interesting from a sociological or community perspective (for example, film or movie sites) but are not relevant to most working definitions of politics and democracy, then in the traditional sense, it would be difficult to reach meaningful conclusions about young users' patterns of engagement. On the other hand, if we were to focus on the websites of traditional political organisations (for example, Parliament, government, political parties or MPs) we may well produce meaningful findings as our material will be political, but those findings may be futile without knowing if and how targeted and potential audiences receive them.

Adapting methodology to the online environment

Taking into account the cultural and technological shifts outlined above, we argue that a research design including web content analysis should acknowledge its variations from traditional content analysis and attempt to accurately and systematically capture the online political message. This can be accomplished on at least three levels.

Epistemological approach

Researchers have now bridged traditional divides between quantitative and qualitative research (Bauer and Gaskell, 2000). One can conduct web content analysis without exclusively adopting a positivistic top-down approach or a totally interpretive, bottom-up one. Qualitative and quantitative inquiries can and should be combined when deemed appropriate. While the mere quantity of web pages and messages offers fertile ground for quantitative analysis, the legitimacy of a statistical sampling process may be questioned. Unless one defines and subsequently analyses an entire population, for example a census such as the Government on the Web 1 and 2 projects (Dunleavy *et al.*, 2002), a more organic, bottom-up approach to sampling is recommended.

There are other ways to use quantitative methodology, for instance through the use of quantitative measurements – variables or categories – such as a word count of various sections, as used by Gibson and Ward (2000). Once again, such measurements can provide useful results, but they should not be treated as the definitive analytical tools. For example, a site very rich in material or containing long paragraphs will not necessarily appeal to younger users whose surfing criteria and attention span may be different from those building the sites. Moreover, web pages containing large galleries of images or other material that extends download time may deter users from visiting. A site using Flash technology may look trendy but it will also be inaccessible to a large number of users whose browsers do not support such functions. Thus, our coding categories (i.e., accessibility, navigation, interaction, content, community) need to acknowledge the preferences of young users.

Methods

We recommend that an ideal research design should combine web content analysis with another method (i.e. triangulation), so that each method can help to overcome the limitations of the other, as well as provide complementary data that builds a more complete picture. While content analysis is a very useful tool that can produce fascinating results about the message itself in general, unaided, it can give us very little information about either the intended impact of a message or its actual use by the users or audiences. This does not reflect a weakness of the medium; rather, it is an essential part of communication. Various communication theories have shown how a message can be distorted or negotiated along its journey from producer to receiver. Unless one actually surveys either the relevant producer or receiver, they can only generate presumptions about that message's intended or actual meaning or effect. Due to the challenges previously discussed in relation to online analyses, it becomes clear that it is necessary to gather this additional information in understanding the full impact of a website.

We point out at least three possible models of triangulation, each consisting of two states of data collection. These models can be adapted and/or mixed into more complex models (Ward and Lusoli, 2003). For a variation of Model 2, see Brady *et al.* (2003).

Model 1

In Model 1, stage 1 consists of a qualitative or quantitative survey or sample of users so as to identify actually visited websites. Stage 2 comprises a content analysis of these relevant websites. This model can provide us with useful information about websites that youth actually visit, and the extent to which they can be considered as political and/or contributing to their engagement. Obviously, utilisation of this model requires us to first define what constitutes a 'political' website. Researchers could either target a specific group of young users or follow up on the findings of an existing survey, such as in research conducted by Ward *et al.* (2005) or those carried out by YouGov.com and the Pew Internet and American Life Project, both of which have provided copies of their questionnaires and data sheets on their websites. Zhao *et al.* (2003) provide another example in their comparative content analysis of Chinese and American websites. They utilise a multi-method research design in that the sampled websites in both countries came from secondary survey data on popular websites.

Model 2

In Model 2, stage 1 includes a content analysis of youth oriented websites, and stage 2 compares the results of the content analysis with users' actual uses/perceptions of those websites. This model differs from the preceding one in that it assesses the effectiveness and take-up of sites that are intended to be facilitating youth civic engagement, as is defined through the sites' own mission statements, content and facilities. As previously mentioned, while analysis of those sites' interaction spaces (for example, chat rooms or message boards) could provide us with useful findings, we assert that the only credible way to judge their impact is by talking to young users themselves. One example of this approach is seen in research performed by Gerodimos (2005). He conducted an in-depth content analysis of UK youth engagement websites and then compared that study's findings, via focus groups, with student users' evaluation. Additionally, Norris (2003) compared the content of party websites ('the supply') with survey data from the websites' users ('the demand').

Model 3

Model 3 incorporates stage 1, a content analysis of youth oriented websites, and stage 2, which complements or compares results of the content analysis with the intended use and content by interviewing webmasters and message producers.

Rather than adopting a user/effects approach, this model can produce comprehensive findings relating to the mission and strategy of a website. As in the second model, we can examine mission statements and written material in determining the intended outreach of the site, and in-depth interviewing provides a higher certainty of an unambiguous understanding of the site's intended meaning. Ward *et al.* (2003) complemented their content analysis of British politics sites with interviews with key personnel, while Jackson (2004) took a relationship marketing approach in comparing the actual output (a content analysis of British political party e-newsletters) with interviews with the e-campaigners of the five parties so as to dissect their political marketing strategy. Singer and Gonzalez-Verez (2003) monitored online newspaper content and also contacted website editors in order to gain more insight into the political aspects of the content.

Sampling

In addition or as an alternative to adopting a qualitative, in-depth case study approach, it is especially important to develop research on networks, which can be conceptualised as vital hosts, carriers and producers of messages. The rise of the Internet has led to the increase in organised networks (Rossiter, 2004) in every aspect of human activity and across a variety of demographic groups. Networks are constituent parts of the Internet not just in terms of hardware, but also in terms of structure, message production, transmission and reception. Whether they be formal or informal, tight or loose, specialised or social, networks are as important to the Internet as traditional institutions are to the physical world, and additionally are an embedded part of young people's life world.

While Hyperlink Network Analysis (HNA) is a dynamically emerging, autonomous branch of Internet studies (Park, 2003), it can and has been combined with content analysis so as to best capture the dynamics of the online world. In support of this line of reasoning, Farrall and Delli Carpini argue that 'given the many and complex dimensions of online discourse, generalizations about the relationship between the Internet and society at large cannot be made from research into single sites and/or by applying single methods' (2004: 287). Using HNA software to trawl co-links among websites, researchers can map social and issue networks online, and then triangulate these results with content analysis of the sites at the core of the network.

Discussion

Content analysis essentially concerns the rigorous study of a political message and provides an in-depth understanding of the product of a communication process. In traditional modes of communication, those messages are finite and easily classifiable in terms of content, space, time and audience/reach. However, the very nature of the Internet and the diffusion of youth culture and communication challenge much of what we know about content analysis. Subsequently, merely transplanting a methodology that has been developed in the context of the old media is not enough to produce a satisfactory analysis of online material.

This chapter has demonstrated that changes in the content, space, time and reach of contemporary political communication and, in particular, those involving young people, force us to update our techniques so as to capture diffused political messages and practices. Possible solutions include: selecting appropriate case studies; using sampling software; incorporating a social networks approach; triangulating content analysis with other methods; and applying a combination of qualitative and quantitative elements.

All four dimensions denote a common trend: that is, the fact that established political processes and institutions are less dominant over the 'political' than they used to be. At the same time, young citizens are at the forefront of a communications revolution with clear effects on the modes of engagement.

The diffusion of content refers to the diffusion of the political into other domains of human activity – cultural, alternative practices and cyber culture, to name a few – which is not a new phenomenon, but is a trend that is both facilitated and accelerated online. Youth culture is central to this shift.

The collapse of space highlights the loss of power by national core executive mechanisms and the problems of legitimation that occur due to the rise of unaccountable transnational policy networks/power centres, but also the potential of civic control of those centres by transnational social movements and grassroots initiatives. In response to this, several scholars have called for international/universal citizenship that would exist in parallel to our currently held nation state nationality, whereas others have noted that the Internet has already risen as an alternative public sphere that challenges dominant and centralised interpretations of political developments (Stevenson, 2000).

The collapse of time marks the increasing role of the global media and the rise of a complex public sphere, as well as a continuous political communication and practice. Youth communication in particular takes place through instant messaging and other means of synchronous interaction and leads to a continuous renegotiation of political expression patterns.

Finally, the pull nature of the Internet aggravates the loss of control by big political organisations and the decline of the dominant narrative within a post-modern virtual space. Traditionally weaker or alternative sources, such as an oppositional blogger, have a greater chance of being heard. Trust in governments, political institutions and established journalists are already declining, especially among the young. The lack of moderation and control over what is transmitted over the Internet has facilitated the explosion of conspiracy theories and differential interpretations.

Thus, the political landscape is changing and traditional democratic institutions need to adapt. In order to develop tools of civic engagement that empower young citizens, we need to capture their online life world not as we are accustomed to imagining it, but as it actually is. As Smith *et al.* (2005: 15) argue, '. . . the key is to recognize that engaging people and organizations in this new environment requires new ways of thinking and new organizational models in order to build a more informed and engaged citizenry'. Web content analysis can be an invaluable tool in that process, but it needs to be distinguished from the methodological constraints of its offline counterpart.

Part II

Making the political connection with young people

9 Technology, schools and citizenship education

A fix too far?

Neil Selwyn

Introduction – a crisis in young people's citizenship?

The last decade or so has seen growing disquiet over social fragmentation, moral decline and rising levels of crime, thus fuelling the perception among many commentators that urgent action is required to re-establish civic stability and, in particular, reconnect young people with society. Indeed, the disconnection between young people and society is seen to be especially pronounced in the area of politics and polity. In the UK it is argued that the post-Thatcher years have been blighted by escalating levels of political apathy and even alienation among the young. This, it is reasoned, has contributed to dwindling electoral turnouts (especially in local government and European elections), plummeting membership of political parties and, most recently, the growth of support for extremist groups such as the British National Party and radical Islam. Thus stark warnings concerning the steady disintegration of civic society have been made, with organisations such as the Electoral Commission (2002) anticipating that 'unless this generation of young people becomes more civic-minded as they age, the nature of British democracy is likely to become increasingly passive'.

Yet this crisis account of modern civic society masks a complex picture of young people and political engagement. On the one hand, young people in Western democracies such as the UK and US are undoubtedly less engaged with formal political processes than preceding generations. As a recent large-scale survey of young people in England and Scotland concluded:

> While young people are interested in social and political issues they do not focus their concerns on engagement with formal political systems. Many hold negative views about politics, such as feeling that they have little control over what the government does.
>
> (Grundy and Jamieson, 2004: 237)

On the other hand there are signs that current generations of young people are *more* civically and politically minded than those in previous decades. Rates of volunteering and charitable donation among young people are reported to be booming, and youth interest and involvement in non-formal and single-issue political causes is similarly high (Roker *et al.*, 1999). As such, it could be contended that young people are not disengaged from politics *per se*, but engaged in ways which are perhaps too informal, fragmented or individualised to contribute to the greater good of formal societal and political structures. As such, it has begun to be recognised that the key challenge faced by the political establishment is not necessarily to politicise a wholly apathetic and apolitical body of young people, but to redirect and remould the young in ways 'appropriate for a democratic and pluralistic society' (Davies *et al.*, 2005(a): 352). This is seen to require the state and wider civic and political communities to somehow increase young people's sense of communitarianism, civic responsibility and obligation, as well as develop their willingness and interest in engaging with formal political and democratic processes.

The turn towards school-based citizenship education

Throughout the 1990s, these concerns prompted a concerted drive in the UK by state and civic stakeholders to seek to redress the apparent political and democratic deficit among young people. Most notably these efforts centred around the championing of a notion of 'citizenship' which drew ideological inspiration from the work of T.H. Marshall (1950). The widespread appropriation in the 1990s of Marshall's view of a rights-based citizenship is not surprising, chiming as it did with the social justice and communitarianism preoccupations of the incoming centre-left Labour administration. Thus, in UK policy circles the overriding aim of fostering citizenship came to be seen in terms of instilling a civil sense of basic rights and protections, political rights (such as voting and public assembly) and rights to social citizenship (such as employment, housing, health care and other social welfare benefits).

From the mid-1990s onwards the UK citizenship project has taken many forms. There has been, for example, a succession of public education campaigns about the need to vote in elections and an ongoing drive to open up the machinations of government to individual citizens. Yet in terms of developing and fostering notions of citizenship among young people, a principal strategy has been that of establishing a national framework of school-based citizenship education. Indeed, the UK government continues to store considerable faith in the social engineering of young citizens through the formal education system (Kerr *et al.*, 2005). As Gordon Brown recently reflected:

> We must address what holds [Britain] back: low turnouts, youth disengagement, falling party membership and a long-term decline in trust – problems that owe more to our political system than our civic culture . . . how, by better citizenship courses in our schools, can we address disengagement among the young?
>
> (Brown, 2006: 32)

As with all innovations in education, this political turn to the classroom is not an especially new or radical phenomenon. Many of the broad elements of the current citizenship drive have long been embedded into teaching and learning in UK schools – either implicitly in disciplines such as English, history and geography, or else under a number of subject titles such as civics, life skills, moral education, personal and social education and character education. Although all taking subtly different approaches to how citizenship can be taught and learnt these subjects have been a long-standing, if often marginalised, feature of schools and schooling over the latter half of the twentieth century (Morris and Cogan, 2001; Arthur and Davidson, 2000).

Yet the version of citizenship education which emerged during the 1990s is distinguished by its forceful positioning as a core and transformatory element of compulsory schooling. This was due in no small part to the involvement of the eminent political scientist Bernard Crick who was tasked by the new Labour government in 1997 with setting up an Advisory Group on citizenship education with a remit to reporting to the UK curriculum and qualifications authority. Crick had been involved in the citizenship debate since the 1970s (for example, Crick, 1978), and his social scientific concerns with formal political participation and communitarianism had considerable bearing on the eventual formalisation of the citizenship curriculum. As such, the eventual Crick Report left the UK with a notion of citizenship education geared towards the ambitious ideals of strengthening formal democracy and creating '"good" citizens [who are] personally responsible, participatory, and justice oriented' (Westheimer and Kahne, 2004: 237). Citizenship education was therefore adopted as a key part of the UK government's strategy to 'encourage greater participation by young people in our democratic life as well as developing the skills they need to prosper socially and economically' (DfEE, 1999).

Thus in 2002 citizenship was formally introduced in England as a foundation subject of the National Curriculum for pupils aged 11 to 16 years, and part of a non-statutory framework alongside Personal Social and Health Education for pupils aged 5 to 11 years. These orders formalised the expectation that young people would gain knowledge and understanding about becoming 'informed' citizens, develop skills of enquiry and com-munication and develop skills of participation and what was termed as 'responsible' action. As such, the revised National Curriculum guidelines for citizenship closely followed the Crick Advisory Group's (1998) identification of three inter-related components of education for citizenship, defined as:

- *social and moral responsibility*: young people learning self-confidence and socially and morally responsible behaviour both in and beyond the classroom, towards those in authority and towards each other;
- *community involvement*: young people learning and becoming helpfully involved in the life and concerns of their neighbourhood and

communities, including learning through community involvement and service to the community;

- *political literacy*: young people learning about institutions, problems and practices of their democracy.

Yet despite its heightened official standing and substantial supporting infrastructure, citizenship education fast assumed a marginal and ineffective place in the actual practice and provision of UK schools. Once the novelty of the Crick Report and the National Curriculum changes faded, considerable concern began to be raised over the peripheral impact of the subject. A succession of reports from the Schools Inspectorate characterised citizenship education as 'marginalised', 'not well established' and even the 'worst taught subject in England' (for example, OfSTED, 2003, 2005; Bell 2005). In particular these inspectorate reports highlighted a lack of effort on the part of schools to reach a 'shared understanding . . . of what citizenship involves' (OfSTED, 2003: 4). As Davies *et al.* (2005a: 354) concluded after the first three years of citizenship education provision, 'the citizenship education initiative in England is very new and somewhat fragile. Training for teachers is limited and school practice is relatively weak.'

As these evaluations imply, much of the 'blame' for the modest showing of citizenship education has been attributed to schools and their teaching staff –replicating a long-standing antagonism in UK education between those responsible for developing curriculum change and those responsible for delivering it. For many educationalists this 'failure' of provision was not wholly unexpected; as Dixon (2000: 94) reflected before the introduction of National Curriculum orders, the 'requirement for schools in Britain to teach citizenship can hardly be said to be response to lively grass roots enthusiasm amongst teachers'. Studies before and after the National Curriculum changes had reported a significant proportion of teachers to perceive citizenship education as a burden (Supple, 1999; Holden, 2004) – a trend felt to have been exacerbated since the introduction of the citizenship curriculum by constraints in terms of resources, time and teacher confidence (Davies, 2006: 5). These school-level issues, it is argued, have led 'many teachers [to be] under-prepared and feel constrained in their ability to handle this aspect of their [citizenship] work' (Oulton *et al.*, 2004), leaving the majority of teaching staff feeling demoralised and restricted in their ability to deliver citizenship education (Schweisfurth, 2006). As such, only a few years after its formal introduction, the UK citizenship education project was seen to have run into significant (some would argue terminal) school-based barriers to achieving its wider aims of reviving the civic and political fortunes of the country.

Aside from the shortcomings of schools and teachers, an equally damning set of criticisms followed the publication of the Crick Report, of the misguided driving ideology of the citizenship curriculum – most notably the observation that the content and approach of citizenship education lacked relevance to young people and society in the early twenty-first century. As Lawy and Biesta have argued:

> The character and complexion of citizenship in Britain has undergone a profound and substantial transformation in the last 50 years. These changes have included the opening up of national borders and the increasing globalisation of the economy and of mass communications technologies. Despite these changes the Marshallian discourse of citizenship has continued to cast a long shadow over contemporary discussion about citizenship policy and practice.
>
> (2006: 36)

In particular the notion of citizenship as it is currently enshrined within the National Curriculum continues to be portrayed by some critics as too narrowly constructed around a passive notion of 'citizenship-as-achievement' instead of a more contemporary notion of 'citizenship-as-practice'. Thus, academic commentators such as Lawy and Biesta have argued that citizenship education in the UK remains outmoded in its privileging of the delivery of information rather than attempting to concentrate on the 'lived experiences' of citizenship-as-practice. This feeling of irrelevance has, therefore, compounded the lack of confidence which built up during the first few years of the 2000s within the educational profession towards citizenship education. If citizenship as a subject is beyond the means of schools and their teachers to deliver effectively, *and* if the citizenship curriculum is of profound irrelevance to the young people it is intended to transform then, it is generally agreed, fundamental change is required if citizenship education is to ever achieve its ambitions of democratic revival.

The turn towards technology-based citizenship education

It is from this background that a growing belief has emerged of late within the citizenship education community that new technologies such as computers, the Internet and video-conferencing can successfully reinvent and reinvigorate the citizenship curriculum. In part, this educational turn towards ICTs derives from wider perceptions that new technology is substantively altering the contemporary political, democratic and civic landscape. As we have seen, technologies such as the Internet are widely seen to be leading to transformed, citizen-centred versions of political and civic engagement. New technologies are seen to be altering issues of political identification, sovereign allegiance and notions of shared culture (Miller, 2001), as well as providing new spaces for political and civic engagement. Many writers have described reconfigured forms of 'digital citizenship' (for example, Black, 1998; Shelley *et al.*, 2004) where the rise of the 'virtual' individual and myriad online communities has substantively changed the manner in which citizens can engage with democracy (Baddeley, 1997; Jordan, 1999). Moreover, technology is seen to be especially pertinent to the citizenship and civic engagement of young people. Indeed, new technologies have been promoted as a particularly 'natural' means of allowing young people to play active roles in society (Garnett, 2005). All told, an 'intrinsically equitable, decentralised and democratic world' (Graham, 2002: 35) is anticipated, with young people technologically repositioned at its core rather than the periphery with 'newfound power' (Montgomery *et al.*, 2004: 125) borne from technology and new media.

Given the assumed centrality of technology to young people's role as citizens in twenty-first century society it is not surprising that ICTs are beginning to be positioned at the heart of the content and delivery of citizenship education. The computer and Internet have been seized upon by some citizenship educators as offering ready solutions to the problem of relevance, as well as overcoming the shortfalls of provision which are seen to have hitherto restricted the citizenship curriculum. Indeed, the affordances of digital technologies for teachers and schools to deliver an effective citizenship curriculum are felt to equal the advantages of their relevance to young people. The ease with which ICTs allow teachers and their students to access ideas, information and people outside the immediate geographical and cultural surroundings of the school is seen by many educators to be reason enough to position them at the centre of the citizenship curriculum (for example, Risinger, 1997).

Much time, effort and funding has been devoted to establishing technology-based citizenship education in the UK, most prominently centring around the use of ICT as a valuable source of citizenship information, as well as the use of ICT as a means of taking part in citizenship discussion and debate. There has been a burgeoning creation of citizenship content for the World Wide Web, a use seen to fit readily with the National Curriculum requirement of helping young people develop 'knowledge and understanding about becoming informed citizens'. Since 2002 government departments, non-governmental organisations, commercial companies and other interest groups have all contributed to the creation of a substantial online presence of citizenship information.

Alongside economies of time, cost and effort, the educational advantages of using ICT in this manner are many – allowing learners and teachers access to a wide range of information, opinions and perspectives from around the world that would otherwise be inaccessible. These online resources have been complemented by the development of a considerable number of citizenship software packages that simulate social situations with the aim of encouraging empathetic discussion and decision making among learners. Typically such software involves the presentation of various scenarios, often in the form of an ongoing narrative, with the learner(s) required to make decisions and judgements at regular intervals which then influence the course of the narrative. The educational appeal of all these resources for citizenship educators is obvious – as Davies *et al.* (2005a: 354) reflected, 'it is clear that teachers will look for easy-to-use resources that are labelled "citizenship"'.

Interest in the use of computer-mediated communication for citizenship education has also grown of late, mirroring general enthusiasm for the use of ICTs to engage young people via online democratic debate. Again, the logic of this use of technology is felt to be sound not least, as Enslin *et al.* (2001: 116) observe: 'talk is obviously fundamental to citizenship' as is listening and cooperating with others, tolerating other points of view and the ability to construct a reasoned argument. If allowed the time and space to talk in school, then students are seen to be capable of expressing sophisticated and complex notions of their cultural identities and status as citizens (for example, Rassool, 1999). From this perspective, the role of ICTs like email and video-conferencing in facilitating and engendering discussion of citizenship matters has been welcomed widely by educators, not least as it corresponds with the National Curriculum strand of 'developing skills of enquiry and communication'. Indeed, one of the few 'ICT opportunities' suggested in the framing National Curriculum documents in 2002 was that 'pupils could use e-mail to exchange views'. Thus, a range of email-based citizenship projects have emerged during recent years, from the British Council-run 'Windows on the World' project to the 'i-learn' organisation's 'learning circles' of students across Africa, South and North America, Australia and the Middle East.

ICT and citizenship education – a fix too far?

These examples, and the many more like them, reflect the increasing amounts of time, funding and effort that are now being devoted to ICT-based citizenship education in the classroom in the hope that it can revitalise the ideals and aims of the government's citizenship project. As such, ICTs have become highly symbolic of the UK citizenship agenda as well as ensuring that 'citizenship' has become a significant element of the multi-million pound schools software marketplace. Given the amount of time, effort and funding now being directed towards ICT-based citizenship education, we would argue that time needs to be taken for some critical reflection as to whether these efforts are likely to be successful or not – both in terms of their educational *and* their political ambitions.

Our cautious approach derives from a notoriously chequered history of educational application of ICTs in schools. In education, as in many other areas of society, there has been a pronounced tendency to embrace new technologies as a panacea to, often, substantial social issues. Much of what is assumed about ICT and education by its proponents stems from a viewpoint where virtually all of society's problems, be they economic, political, social or ethical, are subject to the 'technical fix' of ICT (Volti, 1992) – a deterministic belief which has more often than not failed to be realised. Thus the willingness of education and educationalists to readily appropriate ICTs in such a cause-and-effect fashion should give us sufficient reason to reconsider in more detail the supposed ready solution of ICT-based citizenship education.

Indeed, the potential of ICTs to unproblematically enhance citizenship education in all the ways outlined above can be robustly challenged, raising the less often considered possibility that ICTs may, in fact, do little to alter the inconsistent and ineffectual teaching of citizenship in schools. As Masters *et al.* (2004: 17) contend, it could be the case that 'merely providing online mechanisms is not enough to encourage active citizenship'. For instance, if we reconsider how ICTs are being currently applied to UK citizenship education it is clear that much of the effort to date has sought to use ICTs to reaffirm and augment the official National Curriculum notion of citizenship education. In this way, ICTs are being appropriated to simply repackage and represent existing knowledge, practices and pedagogies in more convenient and palatable forms, without addressing some of the fundamental problems of the citizenship education project. At worst, it could, therefore, be argued that these uses of ICT to technologically replicate the offline citizenship curriculum may contribute to a further deterioration of standards, 'rarely engag[ing] students in anything more than an exchange of information' (Dixon, 2000: 96) and promoting a 'thinner' form of citizenship in terms of the ease with which young people can become politically expressive without being substantively engaged (Howard, 2005). Indeed, one of the few empirical classroom studies of ICT-based citizenship education highlighted the danger of learners developing little real understanding of citizenship issues, with the researchers observing that students were able to repeat stereotyped facts and viewpoints but displayed little deep understanding of the topics involved (McFarlane, *et al.*, 2000). We must, therefore, consider the possibility that increased levels of citizenship information will merely 'create a kind of illusion of being informed . . . not a guarantee of active citizenship, but a substitute for it' (Buckingham, 1999: 174).

Addressing the continuing weaknesses of the citizenship education agenda

We would argue that these concerns should not be discounted as misguided Luddism or conservative knee-jerk reaction to educational innovation. Instead, they raise some potentially fundamental weaknesses of ICT-based citizenship education as it is currently being implemented in UK schools. In particular, the ICT-based citizenship education drive has all the bearings of being a classic technical fix to what was an already dubious 'educational fix' for the perceived political and civic woes of modern society. Thus ICT-based citizenship education finds itself in the weakened position of being a 'fix too far', with technology now being used to compensate for the failings of an education system which itself is being used to compensate for a set of political and societal failings. Indeed, the simplistic view that 'young people will suddenly want to be involved with politics and decision-making because the Internet makes it "trendy"' (Masters *et al.*, 2004: 17) prevails in much of the current provision of citizenship education. Yet the primary problem remains that ICT-based citizenship education does not address the underlying social problems of citizenship education's failure or, indeed, the social problems underlying the presumed citizenship crisis itself. As such, many stakeholders in the current citizenship drive are guilty of being seduced by 'the fetishism of information technology as an intrinsically democratizing or de-democratizing force on societies' (Hand and Sandywell, 2002: 197), causing them to perhaps wilfully overlook some fundamental shortcomings of the citizenship education agenda in the face of presumed technological transformation. Yet we would argue that if time is taken to consider these outstanding issues then it should be possible to identify areas for potential improvement. It is this task to which we turn our attention towards for the remainder of this chapter.

First and foremost, the fact remains that ICT has not altered the essential content or focus of citizenship education as it takes place in the classroom. For better or worse, it is clear that ICTs are currently being employed to deliver essentially the same curriculum in a different form (albeit a form which is assumed to appeal to young people as well as their time- and resource-starved teachers). By repackaging a National Curriculum version of citizenship education in a technological form, most (if not all) of the ICT-based activity to date has not altered the underlying irrelevance of citizenship education to a twenty-first century society where citizenship is a more individualised and actively constructed process. In particular, the form of citizenship education being currently provided through ICTs remains passive and top-down – delivering a 'uniform standard' which is 'done to' young people rather than 'done by' them (Olssen, 2004). Thus the current ICT-enhanced model of citizenship education continues to 'conceptualise young people's citizenship as a desirable "outcome" rather than as a process of transformation' (Lawy and Biesta, 2006: 41), crucially lacking a concern with the full and complete lives of young people, especially the active conditions and processes through which they learn the values of citizenship. If the online citizenship curriculum retains a twentieth-century emphasis on the formal structures of citizenship rather than a more contemporarily relevant notion of the *individual* young citizen then it can be strongly argued that ICT-based citizenship education retains a profound irrelevance to the young people it is intended to be engaging.

Similarly, we would argue that the ICT-based citizenship education agenda suffers from a profound overestimation of the general allure and attraction of ICT to young people – especially the assumption that technology in itself will lend the issue of citizenship a renewed air of relevance. While it is easy to assume that most young people are archetypal 'power users' of ICTs the reality of many young people's engagement with new technologies is often more routine, humdrum and 'normal' (Wagner, 2000). Although Internet applications may well be deeply embedded in the social lives of some young people, for many others the Internet remains a decidedly 'fragile medium', which is used (if at all) in far more limited, sporadic and often conservative ways (Livingstone, 2003). Thus, it is all too easy to misjudge young people's overall enthusiasm and appetite for using ICTs, especially in ways which adults would consider desirable and life-enhancing. Despite the celebration of powerful 'online youth civic cultures' constructed around young people's creation of websites, participation in issue specific forums and maintenance of weblogs (for example, Montgomery *et al.*, 2004), in reality young people's enthusiasm for these technologies is far less prevalent than some commentators would wish to imagine.

We would argue that there is little basis to assume that ICTs will make young people any more engaged with citizenship education or, indeed, any more likely to engage with the formal civic and political processes that are felt to constitute 'citizenship'. Indeed, throughout the citizenship education drive there is an underlying assumption that ICTs can somehow prompt young people to develop profoundly new patterns of engagement and types of activity, propelling young people who have thus far failed to participate in citizenship education to re-engage on their own terms and interests. Yet this logic flies in the face of what we know about ICTs and social inclusion, where a host of empirical studies have found no evidence of such extensions of empowerment. For instance, ICTs have been found to do little to alter patterns of disenfranchisement or abstinence from voting with young adults (Mossberger *et al.*, 2003). Similarly, in terms of political activism and engagement 'there is no sign of the Internet mobilising those who are not already engaged in political activities' (Hargittai, 2004: 140). Thus, rather than prompting those to alter their existing behaviour there are strong grounds to believe that while ICT-based interventions may well be capable of *increasing* levels of citizenship learning and even civic engagement, they will have little impact on *widening* these activities beyond those who were already doing so.

What future for ICT and citizenship education?

Without some fundamental changes it would be reasonable to conclude that ICT-based citizenship education faces something of an impasse. As we have seen, there are strong arguments that fostering a sense of citizenship among young people remains beyond the means of the National Curriculum as it currently stands. There are similarly strong arguments that the current use of new media is doing little to compensate for the restrictions of the school and national curriculum. It is clear that any future schools-based delivery of citizenship education requires significant change, not least a rethinking of what we see as citizenship, politics and civic society in the early twenty-first century, as well as an adjustment in the nature of schools' relationships with knowledge *and* technology. Thus, there is a pressing need for the reconstruction of citizenship education and ICT-based citizenship education around the needs of young people and the realities of contemporary society and citizenship. Resistance to any fundamental reworking of citizenship education is likely to be strong. Recently, Bernard Crick warned against citizenship education being diluted by the 'postmodernism of the streets' (Crick, 2004: 10), but we would argue that this is precisely what is required to revitalise citizenship into a relevant and effective element of contemporary education. As such, rather than starting from the interests and agendas of the formal political establishment, effective citizenship education should 'somehow incorporate or start from that which is already important to the majority of young people' (Supple, 1999: 19). With this in mind we can conclude by discussing how such change may be achieved.

First and foremost, there is a definite need to engineer a change in the nature of formal politics if we are to expect increased engagement from young people. No amount of technological (re)presentation alters the fact that citizenship education is predicated upon 'the same old electoral and institutional politics' (Scammell, 2000: 356). At present there is little to encourage the belief that ICT-based citizenship education will increase young people's engagement or interest. As Stephen Coleman (2005b: 33) has argued, 'even when transmitted by the most sophisticated and cutting-edge multi-media technologies, dull political messages are still dull political messages and grey politicians are still just as miserably grey'. From this perspective, there is a need for practitioners and politicians to avoid seeing increased access to citizenship information and resources via media as somehow leading to increased levels of citizenship and, instead, seek to address the serious shortcomings of the political system. This is, of course, not an easy task but it would seem essential to move away from the 'essentially orthodox agendas' that currently hold little resonance with today's young people (Davies and Issitt, 2005).

Aside from this rather idealistic call for the widespread reinvention of formal politics, there are some more practicable signs as to how the scope of citizenship as it currently is laid out within the National Curriculum can be broadened beyond the concerns of the formal political establishment. In particular, it would seem sensible that the 'citizenship curriculum' which is delivered in schools recognises the emergence of new forms of citizenship at a time when the modern social contract is undergoing a process of transformation (Magalhães and Stoer, 2003). For example, it has been persuasively argued that citizenship is now less determined by links to national identity and nationally determined sets of rights and duties than structured through other local and global identities. One's political identity and awareness can now be rooted in a village, a city, a region, a country, a continent, one's sexuality or (as is prevalent in the lives of many young people) patterns of consumption. Many political and social scientists are beginning to argue that democratic citizenship now derives less from a political public than from a 'civic public' rooted in ideas about the freedom to consume through the logic of privatisation (Lukose, 2005). It can be strongly argued that the act of consuming entails a civic duty, public-spiritedness and self-education that conventional notions of citizenship are built around. Thus, as Scammell (2000: 351) argues:

> The act of consumption is becoming increasingly suffused with citizenship characteristics and considerations. Citizenship is not dead, or dying, but found in new places, in life-politics, as Anthony Giddens calls it, and in consumption. The site of citizens' political involvement is moving from the production side of the economy to the consumption side. As workers, most of us have less power now for all the familiar reasons . . . As consumers, though, we, at least in the developed North, have more power than ever.
>
> (Scammell, 2000, p. 351)

Thus a citizenship curriculum that at least entertains the idea that citizenship for most young people may not equate with being citizen-workers or citizen-voters but perhaps citizen-consumers or citizen-lifestylers would achieve a relevance and appeal to young people that has hitherto eluded it. If the content of the citizenship curriculum can be expanded to reflect the fact that citizenship is changing in these more informal ways then, we would contend, citizenship education may achieve the relevance it has otherwise lacked to date.

As well as altering the content and ideological approach of citizenship education there is also a clear need to alter the ways in which schools operate with regards to their relationships with information and knowledge, as well as their appropriation of technology. In both instances this involves schools and teachers feeling comfortable to draw on the knowledge and technological practices of their students, thus off-setting their own deficiencies in expertise and resourcing as well as increasing the relevance to young people of what takes place in the classroom. For example, it would seem sensible that schools make more use of the knowledge and processes inherent in the formation of young people's citizenship outside of the school in different contexts and at various places in the local community. As Lawy and Biesta note, 'young people routinely participate in a range of different [citizenship] practices such as the family, peers, school and college, leisure, work and the media. These provide qualitatively different opportunities for action and hence qualitatively different opportunities for learning-from-action' (2006: 45). Thus citizenship education inside the school would be enhanced by recognising and drawing upon these outside-school knowledges and practices instead of resisting or denying them. Instead of young people having to 'check in their local knowledges' before entering the classroom (McNeill, 1988) a reinterpretation of the relationship between school and community is required 'that suggests that this relationship should not only be sensitive to but even porous with regard to local knowledges and sociabilities' (Magalhães and Stoer, 2004: 329). In theory, schools and teachers should be striving to draw upon the citizenship knowledges and practices of their students, with young people being allowed to bring all of themselves into schools (Audigier, 1998).

Finally, we would argue that citizenship education would be further improved by a 'bottom-up' approach to schools' relationships with, and appropriations of, technology. Reflecting the individually-focused notion of citizenship there is a clear need for schools to allow an individually-driven use of ICTs, rather than the school-controlled and often restricted use of technologies which currently characterises much ICT use in the classroom. This would entail a move away from 'the strict organisational and curriculum use' of ICTs in the form of officially-produced web pages, simulation software, staged email exchanges and the overriding concern with only allowing access to material considered 'suitable' and not 'anarchic' (Kendall, 2000: 6).

Schools have been rather poor in allowing young people to use ICTs as they wish, but the increased personalisation and mobility of ICTs is seeing a shift away from centrally managed systems to devices and resources managed and controlled by young people, which they bring from home to school. It is clear that school systems and infrastructure need to respond to these new approaches, altering the ways in which school-based learning is managed and controlled to allow greater flexibility and more fluidity between different sites of learning and different systems (Selwyn, 2003). Although this is generally seen as a profound challenge to schools, it could also be seen as an opportunity for an area of the curriculum like citizenship education. For example, it has been widely argued that young people should be able to freely create their own citizenship material, rather than merely passively consuming pre-existing content. As Buckingham (1999: 182) persuasively argues:

> If the struggle for citizenship is partly a struggle over the means and substance of cultural expression – and particularly over those which are made available by the electronic media – it is essential that the school curriculum should enable young people to become actively involved in the media culture that surrounds them. From this perspective [we should] encourage young people's critical participation as cultural producers in their own rights.

Conclusion

In this chapter we have attempted to sketch out a reworking of ICT-based citizenship education where both the content of the citizenship curriculum and the application of new technologies is more individually focused and determined. Yet at present it would be fair to conclude that many of the problems faced by citizenship education are not necessarily amenable to a quick 'technical fix' but instead require a more fundamental rethink of what citizenship is in the early twenty-first century. Only by reorientating the presently rather rigid citizenship curriculum towards the more fluid and individualised realities of twenty-first century citizenship, can citizenship education achieve the relevance and dynamism it currently seeks through the application of ICTs. Whereas new technologies have a role to play in enabling this individualisation and bottom-up reshaping, ICTs alone cannot be expected to revitalise the citizenship curriculum – this is something that requires profound educational and political change.

Of course, while citizenship education can be improved in the ways outlined in this chapter, the outcomes of any form of citizenship education are unlikely to ever satisfy the ambitions of the governments that implement them. As such, the citizenship potentials of technology should not be used as a distraction to the considerable burden of expectation being placed upon schools and teachers to act as a 'fix' to the wider problems of society. Thus, it is important for all stakeholders to recognise that the fostering of engaged young citizens is not just an educational responsibility. As Lawy and Biesta (2006: 47) conclude, 'responsibility for citizenship should not be confined to schools and colleges, nor should it rest with teachers or the structuring of the curriculum. It is a responsibility that extends to society at large.' Thus, our recommendations for change notwithstanding, there is a concurrent responsibility on the political elite to refocus their approach to citizenship education away from one of an easy 'political fix' to being just one element in a wider effort to reconcile formal politics and current generations of young people. This is something that technology and schools cannot be expected to achieve on their own.

10 Reconnecting young people in Northern Ireland

Roger Austin

This chapter is concerned with the role of ICT in citizenship education in Northern Ireland. The main argument presented here is that the evolution of thinking about citizenship in the curriculum has taken relatively little account of the role that ICT might play in enabling schools in a divided society to work together. It is further argued that unless the concepts of intercultural competence and re-schooling are fully understood, the opportunities for reconnecting young people will be very limited. The first section sets the context through an analysis of the political and educational situation in the period since the 1998 Good Friday peace agreement. The second offers a critique of citizenship education in the curriculum, and the third examines the ways in which ICT has been used to re-connect young people.

Political and educational context

Northern Ireland has a population of 1.9 million of whom an estimated 40,000 are non-Caucasian; their relatively small numbers have not until recently impacted on perceptions of citizenship, which continue to be dominated by matters of social and political identity. Northern Ireland is the place where the United Kingdom and the Republic of Ireland meet and where there continue to be strongly held views about whether its people are 'British', 'Irish' or 'Northern Irish'.

It is a part of the United Kingdom that has been marked by severe inter-communal violence in the period from 1968 to 1997. Although the Good Friday Agreement of 1998 marked a significant step in the recent history of Northern Ireland in terms of reducing the level of political violence, mutual suspicion between the locally elected political parties has meant that power sharing between the unionist camp and the Nationalist/ Republican camp has had limited success. Since 2002, the failure of local political representatives to be able to govern, has led to a resumption of 'direct rule' (Northern Ireland Office, 2006).[1]

In effect, politicians elected in England, Scotland or Wales are appointed by the British prime minister to administer Northern Ireland. Citizenship education in Northern Ireland is therefore operating in an unusual setting where, for example, the generally accepted principles of democratic representation are played out in a very different way to what exists in England, Scotland and Wales. The people of Northern Ireland elect representatives to local councils and MPs to the Parliament in Westminster but the suspension of the Northern Ireland assembly means that many decisions, in health, education and housing, are taken by ministers who are not accountable to the electorate in Northern Ireland. Furthermore, social policy decisions have to be seen in the wider context of security issues and of long-term British strategic objectives in Northern Ireland.

The body politic in Northern Ireland is also strikingly different to the rest of the United Kingdom in terms of the composition and outlook of the political parties that campaign in local, Westminster or European elections. None of the main Westminster-based political parties, Labour, Liberal Democrat and Conservative, campaign in Northern Ireland; instead, voters are offered political choices which reflect different strands of Unionism through the Democratic Unionist party or the Ulster Unionist party, or Republicanism and Nationalism through Sinn Fein and the Social Democratic and Labour Party, both of which aspire to a united Ireland. The only other political parties, which campaign on the basis that they are not sectarian, the Alliance party, the Green party and the Women's Coalition,[2] attract very few votes. In effect, the unresolved constitutional question about whether Northern Ireland is 'British' or 'Irish' continues to dominate political discourse. So when we talk about what citizenship education means in Northern Ireland, we cannot ignore the political reality that whatever benefits there have been from the reduction of violence since 1997, the price that was paid when a power sharing executive was set up, was a strengthening of the traditional local parties whose constituents often vote according to historical and religious allegiance. In effect, Northern Ireland remains a deeply divided society with divisions that permeate almost every aspect of daily life.

As recently as March 2005, an influential government document called 'A Shared Future' (OFM, 2005) published by the Secretary of State for Northern Ireland, referred to 'communal polarisation' and to the 'economic and social imperative of tackling the costs of division'. While it asserted that government aims were to 'build a shared, tolerant and inclusive society', and that 'separate but equal' was not an option, the report accepted that in reality, inter-communal tensions meant that the provision of 'parallel services' for the two main groups in society, broadly Protestant and Catholic, was commonplace. The report noted that this was particularly true for education where only 55 schools, representing some 5 per cent of the school population, were formally 'integrated'. In addition to the choice that parents have in terms of whether they send their children to a 'controlled' school (state funded and influenced by the Protestant churches), a maintained school where the influence of the Catholic church would be marked, or an integrated school where children from diverse backgrounds are educated together, there are further divisions between grammar schools, which recruit on the basis of performance in an 11+ examination and secondary schools which do not. The direct rule government has decided that the 11+ examination will be discontinued from 2008 and that selection to a post-primary school may not be done on the basis of academic performance.

In addition to the choice of schools already described, the Northern Ireland administration has agreed to support a small number of Irish medium primary and post-primary schools. The net result of this policy, coupled with a decline in student numbers, has been both intense competition for students in post-primary schools and a view that there are too many small schools that will find it difficult to deliver the broad range of academic and vocational subjects to students from the age of 14. The government's dilemma is that while the existing diversity of secondary school provision suits the principle of parental choice, it is expensive to the UK tax payer and it reinforces the social and denominational divisions. School amalgamation or closure is likely to be fiercely resisted by parents and the main churches, supported by local political parties who have shown little support for schooling solutions that bring children together under one roof.

The curriculum

The government's approach to these difficulties has been to limit the effect of differences between school ethos by insisting that there should be a common curriculum followed by all schools and that parts of the curriculum should specifically address the divisions within Northern Ireland and beyond. In 'A Shared Future' (2005), it is argued that between 1995 and 2005 there have been a number of important educational developments towards a 'more inclusive society'. Specific reference is made to the cross-curricular themes of Education for Mutual Understanding (EMU) and Cultural Heritage (CH) introduced in 1989, and to the inter-school links funded through the School Community Relations Programme which began in 1987 (O'Connor *et al.*, 2002). The report asserts that 'in the revised curriculum shortly to be implemented, these themes will continue as integral parts of the citizenship programme' (2002: 26). It is intended that citizenship, at present an optional part of the curriculum, will become mandatory from September 2007; the significant status given to citizenship sits in sharp contrast to the rest of the curriculum where the focus is less on 'subjects' and much more on the development of skills. To explain this paradox, we need to understand how citizenship, with its emphasis on conceptual understanding of key ideas, has eclipsed the cross-curricular themes of Education for Mutual Understanding and Cultural Heritage.

At the centre of much EMU and cross-community school work was the notion that the 'contact hypothesis', drawing on research in social psychology, would improve relationships between different groups if certain conditions of contact were met. Crucially, it was suggested that successful contact was more likely to occur if the contact was between people of equal status, based on cooperation rather than competition, was long term rather than short term, had a clear agreed goal and was backed by institutional support (Allport, 1954). However, the translation of these precepts into working practice in Northern Ireland came into question in the mid-1990s; Smith and Robinson's 1996 research (Smith and Robinson, 1996) into the impact of EMU suggested that there was little empirical evidence to support the belief that greater contact between groups was likely to lead to a reduction in conflict.

Three later reports, one produced by the Education and Training Inspectorate in 2000 on Education for Mutual Understanding (ETI, 2000) and another on the School Community Relations Programme written by researchers at the University of Ulster for the Department of Education in 2002 (O'Connor *et al.*, 2002), signalled concerns about the effectiveness of EMU and the operation of the cross-community contact scheme. In particular, the 2002 report spoke of a lack of a coherent definition of community relations, deficiencies in training and 'unpurposeful and/or inconsistent school links'. The report also referred to research by Cairns and Hewstone (2001) which suggested that existing contact schemes between schools were not reaching young people with sectarian attitudes. Finally, the Chief Inspector's report for the period 2002–04 noted that only 21 per cent of primary school children had taken part in such schemes and that a mere 3 per cent of pupils in post-primary schools had been involved.

The cumulative effect of this research was to lead to a view that every child in Northern Ireland should have a structured learning experience of citizenship as a central element in a revised Northern Ireland curriculum. While the UK government had been developing plans for the introduction of citizenship in the curriculum (Crick, 1998) across the United Kingdom since 1998, what emerged in Northern Ireland had a distinctive character.

The citizenship curriculum in Northern Ireland

After widespread consultation, the Northern Ireland Council for Curriculum, Examinations and Assessment (NICCEA) put forward proposals for a reform of the curriculum (CCEA, 2003) in 2003 which was designed to enable pupils to develop as individuals and as contributors to society, the economy and the environment. A key part of an area of the curriculum called 'Learning for Life and Work', Local and Global Citizenship was to be introduced for the first time around the four key concepts of Diversity and Inclusion, Human Rights and Responsibility, Equality and Social Justice and Democracy and Active Participation. Schools were invited to take part in citizenship education on a voluntary basis from 2003 but, unusually, all post-primary schools were asked to nominate four or five teachers for training from 2004. Only training in ICT had received such a high profile before this, a clear sign of how much importance was attached to this by the Department of Education in Northern Ireland. An interim evaluation of the impact of this work in 2004/5 was published by Niens and O'Connor (2005) based on data collected in 30 schools.

Among the many findings of this detailed report, of particular relevance for this chapter were the very limited extent of cross-community contact between pupils and the equally restricted use of ICT in the pupils' experience of citizenship education. The authors noted that 'large percentages of respondents claimed that none of their relatives (53 per cent), friends (53 per cent) and neighbours (38 per cent) was from the other religious community' (p. 23). Later they note that 'pupils' evaluations of intergroup relations deteriorated significantly over the course of the year' (p. 28). Elsewhere, the report notes that 'pupils from integrated schools reported more learning about sectarianism and conflict resolution' (p. 4) than pupils in controlled or maintained schools. In effect, therefore, while the authors note 'significant and consistent increases in pupils' confidence relating to a variety of behaviours associated with local and global citizenship' (p. 3) these changes occurred for 95 per cent of pupils in largely mono-cultural settings. It prompts the authors to suggest that 'inter-school collaboration might be a useful tool to share good practice between schools'.

We referred earlier in the chapter to the 2005 government policy proposals contained in 'A Shared Future'. This document asserts that in addressing the communal polarisation that they identify as a central problem, and which is also reflected in the interim report on citizenship education, 'relationships are central'. It is clear that whatever good work is being done in schools through citizenship – a subject that is due to become mandatory from September 2007 – the relationships that are being nurtured are primarily with pupils from a similar background. In the following section we examine the ways in which ICT is already being used in Northern Ireland to break this circle by enabling 'virtual' links to be forged between schools.

ICT, citizenship and cross-border links

Since 1986, the Department of Education in Northern Ireland has been promoting both the use of ICT for links between schools and, since the late-1990s, a strategic plan called Classroom 2000 to provide all schools with broadband connectivity and regularly 'refreshed' hardware and software. In this section we offer a critique of the work done to date and seek to explain why the pioneering work carried out has rarely involved links between schools within Northern Ireland.

In 1985, Prime Minister Margaret Thatcher saw the need to look at Northern Ireland in the wider context of relationships between Ireland and the UK. The Anglo-Irish Agreement, signed that year with Irish premier

Garret Fitzgerald, recognised the importance of improving relations between London, Belfast and Dublin and of promoting steps that would help to break down barriers and mistrust. Although the original motivation for this political initiative was to address the short-term problems that had emerged after the IRA hunger strikes of the early 1980s, it was certainly true that ever since the partition of Ireland in 1921, there had been limited cross-border contact.

Along with a number of other initiatives, an educational project was set up in 1986 called the European Studies (Ireland and Great Britain) Project, which was originally designed to use ICT to enable schools in England, Northern Ireland and the Republic of Ireland to work together. The title of the project was unusual, particularly given Thatcher's very public opposition to any suggestion that Europe should intrude on the sovereign rights of the nation state. But the title was well chosen, in that it enabled all parties to explore relationships under the 'safe' umbrella of Europe. As students involved in the project came to realise, being part of the wider European Union family provided an additional level of European citizenship in which you did not have to stop being Irish or British.

The part played by ICT was also significant; this project was one of the first to recognise the role that email, computer conferencing and video-conferencing might play[3] in providing the means for pupils at school to carry out joint investigations of curricular topics across national boundaries. (Austin, 1992a, 1992b, 1992c). Although the term citizenship was not used in any part of this programme, the project clearly intended that through the process of working together towards an agreed goal, pupils should come to understand both similarities and differences of culture within the islands of Great Britain, Ireland and the European mainland.

Furthermore, it was difficult to argue against the proposition that government money should be used on ICT when there was so much emerging evidence about the relationship between ICT investment and productivity (Barber, 2001). This message had a particular resonance in Northern Ireland where even in 2006, it was estimated that 60 per cent of the working population was employed in the public sector. Developing a strong ICT skills base in education was, therefore, a necessary part of promoting an entrepreneurial culture which would enable a region on the geographical periphery of Europe to remain competitive in a global economy.

It says something about the effectiveness of the approach adopted by the European Studies Project that it has continued to flourish, albeit with different sources of funding; whereas at the start of its life from 1986 to 1992, it received government support from London, Belfast and Dublin, it now relies on subventions from Belfast, Dublin and the EU. The withdrawal of financial assistance from London may be seen as an example of the UK government's strategy of cutting back on its financial commitments while also encouraging strong north–south intergovernmental cooperation between Belfast and Dublin.

Dissolving boundaries

Further evidence of the ways that ICT might be used to sustain cross-border educational links can be seen in the work of the Dissolving Boundaries programme set up in 1999 and funded by the Departments of Education in Belfast and Dublin. This programme is important for four reasons.

First, it has been able to demonstrate that ICT can be used effectively for inter-school work with children as young as 9 years of age and those with moderate or severe special educational needs. The project team, based in the University of Ulster and the National University of Ireland, Maynooth, has reported at length on how teachers and pupils have used video-conferencing and computer conferencing to develop joint curricular work (Austin *et al.*, 2003). This has happened in spite of the significant differences between educational structures, the curriculum and teaching conditions in Northern Ireland and the Republic of Ireland. Much of the earlier work carried out in this field had been with pupils in secondary schools and had been largely based on text-based interaction (Austin, 2006); video-conferencing, supported by easy to use videophones operating over ISDN telephone lines, has transformed this picture. The advent of broadband technologies will make video-conferencing cheaper and more accessible.

Second, Dissolving Boundaries has successfully introduced a methodology for joint work through ICT based on small teams in each school working collaboratively with a team of a similar size in their partner school. The combined team work together to investigate an issue and to present their conclusions through presentational software or the creating of a joint web-site. Examples of this can be found on the Dissolving Boundaries website.[4] The successful operation of the programme depends on the willingness of teachers to jointly plan the work and review progress at two annual face-to-face conferences.

Third, this work has had a marked effect on the attitudes and skills of the pupils involved, in terms of an increased sense of self-esteem, improved communications skills and in terms of their views about pupils on the other side of the border. The most recent published evaluation of the work carried out in 2004 (Austin *et al.*), based on teacher and pupil comment, suggests that virtual contact is slowly breaking down barriers. 68 per cent of teachers overall (n = 70) rated the impact of Dissolving Boundaries on north–south understanding as very significant or significant. There were some differences between teachers in the different types of school; 75 per cent of teachers in primary school said that the effect of the project was either very significant or significant in terms of 'north–south understanding', the figure for teachers in special schools was 60 per cent, while for those in post-primary schools it was 62 per cent. These findings are particularly important in the context of the previously quoted negative data about the effect of 'contact' between young people. It may be that greater clarity about overall aims coupled with effective external support for schools has created the conditions in which contact can, indeed, make a difference.

Finally, the funding of the programme by government departments in Belfast and Dublin indicates a growing acceptance of the shared responsibility for addressing persistent cross-border mistrust through purposeful educational links (Pollak, 2006). Where earlier cross-border links were 'wrapped up' in the European dimension, Dissolving Boundaries is one of a number of government or internationally funded schemes that directly address historic cross-border divisions and differences.

One final point should be made at this juncture; during the 1980s and 1990s, innovative use of technology to form school partnerships for language work in Europe, and for links to the USA and Japan showed that there was no lack of interest in connecting young people in Northern Ireland to the wider world (Martin, 2000; Anderson, 2006). Indeed, it is estimated that as many as 50 per cent of post-primary schools in Northern Ireland had some experience of using ICT to forge links that could be seen as supporting global citizenship. We turn next to consider how far this experience has been used for local citizenship between schools within Northern Ireland.

ICT between schools in Northern Ireland

Research into the use of ICT for inter-cultural education has shown that geographical proximity/distance is a significant variable (Sundberg, 2001); in other words, it can be easier to use technology to link to schools far away than those nearer to home where previous conflict or competition for pupils are just two complicating factors. This chapter so far has underlined that the technology to support inter-school links in Northern Ireland has been provided in every school through the development of an overall strategic approach to ICT, delivered through the Classroom 2000 programme. Furthermore, although there are critics of online political discussion who argue that its anonymity simply encourages the use of invective, Coleman in Crick (1998) has a persuasive counter argument:

> On-line discussions offer people a sense of not simply hearing about or being spectators of civic affairs, but becoming involved as deliberating participants. The commonly-stated claim that 'nobody cares what I think' is countered by the ease with which citizens can have their say on-line and experience a sense of being heard and meeting responses; [it] allows citizens to become familiar with the rules (implicit as well as formal) of democratic debate.
>
> (Crick, 1998, Appendix B)

However, there has been very limited use of ICT since 1998 to link schools across the community divide within Northern Ireland. Three initiatives took place between 1998 and the end of 2000 at a time when there was still a measure of optimism around the power-sharing executive that had been set up as part of the Good Friday Agreement. The first involved 73 pupils aged 16–17 in an equal number of Protestant and Catholic schools in May 1998. Student teachers in these schools acted as mentors and moderators of the online discussion, which included questions on the highly controversial early release of both Republican and Loyalist prisoners. The discussion was designed to clarify views in advance of the referendum which gave voters in Northern Ireland the opportunity to endorse or reject the Good Friday Agreement. Analysis of the transcript of the discussion highlights three important points about the use of ICT for links within Northern Ireland.

First, at its best, this kind of interaction is based on critical and well-informed commentary; in response to messages of outrage about the morality of giving early release to prisoners who had committed acts of murder, one contributor noted:

> I think a number of points have to be made concerning the prisoners issue. Firstly, prisoners in NI have benefited for well over a decade from a penal system which is significantly more lenient than that in Britain (or the Republic of Ireland). 408 'life' prisoners have now been released (having served sentences between 11–20 years) as a result of the lifers' release scheme which began in 1984 with the support of all parties. Criticism of this scheme has been conspicuous by its absence . . . Secondly, I'm not sure that it is appropriate for the 'No' camp to repeatedly raise the issue of victims. This is a very emotive issue designed to engender anti-agreement feeling. What they are conveniently ignoring is that many of the victims who they repeatedly fling in our faces are pro-agreement. It must sicken these true victims to have their status/position abused in such a manner.

This response prompted a comment from a representative of one of the political parties, an interesting early indication of the readiness of political representatives to reach out to young people in 1998:

> The fear generated by the prospect of violent prisoners on early release is understandable but the evidence shows that:
>
> - less than 1 per cent of prisoners who had served a life sentence in Northern Ireland re-offend;
> - since 1991 over 9,000 people have served time in prison for scheduled offences. Of these, over 8,500 have already been released; about 400 prisoners currently in prison already qualify for early release. All but 63 of these would have been released anyway within two years;
> - a form of early release has been in operation in Northern Ireland since 1985 under the Life Sentence Review Board.

To claim that this is a critical new issue arising out of the Agreement and one which justifies a 'no' vote in the referendum is quite simply dishonest.

Second, this small-scale project recognised the need to provide mentoring for moderating online discussion though the involvement and tutoring of student teachers, a point that had been well made by Coleman in 1998:

> Some thought is currently being given to the need for training in monitoring on-line democratic discussions. It is necessary to refine these skills and produce 'best practice' guides for moderated interactive discussion. In acquiring these skills, young people could learn much about debating protocols and the importance of developing tolerant approaches to discussion based upon 'hearing' as well as 'speaking'.

One of the reasons why computer conferencing is a particularly valuable medium for the discussion of emotive issues is that it is asynchronous. In other words, participants have time to reflect on what they want to say, can compose responses off-line, and discuss them with fellow pupils and with their teacher before posting them to make them 'live'. Rather than posting in messages direct to a conference, with the attendant risks of spelling or grammar mistakes and ill-considered content, the offline preparation of responses allows considered debate to take place within the class about the propriety of language or content. This at once transforms the context from individual, privately composed opinion, to group and class-mediated views and it avoids casting the teacher as censor or embarrassing a school.

Finally, this case study raises questions about the importance of written communication for effective discussion and highlights a risk of creating a new 'digital divide' between those who struggle with written expression, more often boys than girls according to Millard (1997), and those who do not.

This issue is particularly well illustrated in the second case study which was based around a Bill of Rights Youth Conference and reported on by Milliken (2001). Over a three-day period, online debate took place between handicapped students, young people from both sides of the community, representatives from political parties and the Chief Commissioner of the Northern Ireland Human Rights Commission. Moderation of the conference was entrusted to five young people who were given some training for this role. Significantly, the conferencing software was designed to limit to some 30 words the amount of text that could be sent. Milliken acknowledged that this had 'drawbacks with respect to the depth of discussion permitted', but noted benefits too. The youth moderators commented that the politicians 'couldn't get away with the crap they normally come out with 'cos the system wouldn't let them write long sentences' (Milliken, 2001). Typical exchanges, with participants writing through their own online aliases about the decommissioning of weapons were:

Jonnymckee: what about the guns?

Static 2001:   If guns are handed over they can easily be bought again, what difference will it make?

JOEBANS: FORGET ABOUT THE GUNS THEY ARE SILENT.

Alliancegerry: An SF (SinnFein) activist once said to me, the guns are there for a purpose, even if they are not being fired.

Static2001:   WELL SAID, JOEBANS.

Jonnymckee: a silent gun to my head is still scary.

Static2001:   but no one is holding a silent gun to your head.

Alliancegerry: that's not what a lot of people feel, static. a lot of people feel they can't trust IRA/UDA/UVF- not necessarily me but a lot of people genuinely worry.

JOEBANS: SPEAK FOR YOURSELF, GERRY.

Static 2001:   but will decommissioning really stop the worry, what it all comes down to is the fact that those paramilitaries involved in the talks have cooperated with everything else.

This excerpt shows that informal language, close to the style and format of text messages sent between mobile phones, can still enable an exchange of opinion and, indeed, is one of the fastest growing forms of communication between young people. There is a difficult choice here between encouraging young males to express opinion in a written form using language that does not meet normal 'school' standards of literacy, and insisting on literate responses that might deter the very pupils who should be discussing these issues. Milliken (2001) uses the terms 'empowerment and enfranchisement' to describe key benefits of online conferencing. So, if it is argued that online conferencing is a powerful tool to enable an exchange of informed opinion, ways must be found to marry the spontaneity of the text message with the need for reflective and well-documented exchanges. If this fails, significant sections of the youth population may feel excluded from what they perceive to be an academic and thus inaccessible form of discourse.

The final case study, called the 'On-line with Schools project' took place in November 2000 at a time when a power-sharing executive had been set up following voter support for the Good Friday Agreement. As part of a commitment to open government and to illustrate readiness to embrace the concept of e-government, the Deputy First Minister suggested that a project be set up to allow him 'to connect to schools in Northern Ireland and engage in meaningful dialogue'.

Student teachers were again invited to support the project, but with pupils three to four years younger than in the 1998 study. Furthermore, the schools involved were drawn from the non-selective school sector, where many pupils would not have been successful in the 11+ examination.

Sixteen secondary schools took part and, in the ten days that the online conference was 'live', 194 messages were posted into the conferencing area of the Northern Ireland Network for Education (NINE), the Northern Ireland node of the National Grid for Learning (NGfL). At the end of the online discussion, the Deputy First Minister had a live video-conference link with two participating schools.

In a significant number of respects, this project was different to the other two described so far; first, where the 1998 projects addressed potentially divisive issues directly, the On-Line with Schools Project approached them in a much more oblique manner. For example, in response to the question about what Northern Ireland would be like in ten years' time, the pupils were almost equally divided between those expressing optimism and others who were less hopeful:

> I hope . . . that there will be peace in Northern Ireland, I know I might be a bit ambitious in hoping for [this] but it would be nice to stop all the murders and all the bombs and all the arguing that is going on. What do you think it will be like?
>
> In ten years time life in NI will be the equivalent to the ghettoes of Detroit city as it's becoming a horrible place to live in . . . I don't see a bright future for this country unless Catholics and Protestants can work together and bring back the peace we once had. But I don't think that this will happen as certain politicians have stripped us of any hope of peace by giving us ideas that we should hate each other because of religion.

While these comments were on the record and, therefore, available for all participants to read and respond to, the locus of discussion was generated through questions suggested by the Deputy Prime Minister. The effect of this was to restrict the amount of pupil–pupil exchange but it did not stop some of them from expressing their frustration at being excluded from the political process. Typical comments from both Catholic and Protestant pupils were:

> We feel excluded from politics because we are not old enough to vote. The news is not aimed at young people and we find the political arrangements difficult to understand. We think that schools should provide us with the knowledge of how to be part of the political system so that we can have an input into our future, especially when educational issues are in the news.
>
> As a fourth year student I think there should be more information given to young people like myself. Yes, the political situation of Northern Ireland is never off the television, but the reports assume we understand all that has gone on before. I have started to take an interest in politics as I have got older but I would need a greater knowledge

of the background to the situation as it is now. What do you suggest I and others in my position should do?

The second way in which this case study differed from the previous ones, was the way that these 13- to 15-year-olds seized the opportunity to get outside conventional Northern Ireland political issues and concentrate on what they felt was important. A significant number of comments were posted on what was seen as the inequity of the 11+ examination. In a remarkably prescient comment, one pupil observed:

> The 11+ maybe isn't such a good idea, as it puts a lot of strain on children who want to go to grammar school. I always wanted to go to my High school, so I didn't feel the pressure of 'failing'. I did the 11+ and got an 'A' and I think that this is because I didn't feel pressurised. My point is that many children are pushed and if they fail they think they have let their parents down . . . Children should be 'chosen' into schools based on the work they have done in all of primary school, instead of one test which can 'make or break' a future.

In fact, the present administration decided in 2005 to scrap the 11+ and replace it with precisely the kind of scheme suggested by this pupil. Other comments showed that issues to do with equality were high on the agenda of some of the female participants: 'There should be equal rights in school. Girls should be allowed to wear trousers, I don't see what the difference is. It's very sexist that we aren't allowed to keep warm.' While for others, it was the burden of school bags that mattered most:

> In my school at present there are pupils carrying bags that weigh over a stone in weight. I have been one of those pupils who have had to carry such items as a school bag, PE bag, a musical instrument and after school activities all in the one day. I believe schools should be given more money to place lockers for all pupils as it has been shown in research that carrying a heavy bag is very bad for your back.

What these examples show, is that issues of immediate concern to school pupils can clearly be raised and debated online . . . and these issues are about pupil rights in the broadest sense of that term.

In concluding this section on the use of ICT for links within Northern Ireland, two points are worth underlining. The first is that all the work described in the preceding section was carried out on the margins of the curriculum; it was voluntary and preceded the introduction of citizenship education in the curriculum. Second, there has been relatively little work done between 2000 and 2006 on the use of ICT in citizenship between schools in Northern Ireland and this reflects in part a sharpening of the political landscape with voter preferences going to the less conciliatory

Democratic Unionist Party and Sinn Fein. In such a setting it can be very difficult for teachers to put their heads above the parapet and promote cross-community dialogue, even through ICT.

Conclusion

What conclusions might be drawn from this work that have relevance beyond the shores of the island of Ireland? The first is that the use of ICT for reconnecting young people, especially in a citizenship context carries with it a significant weight of 'values'; there has been relatively little discussion about what values, if any, are associated with particular applications of ICT (Austin, 2004). In our analysis, ICT for the purposes of supporting links between schools is contributing to the broad citizenship agenda, both locally and globally. It does this not by predetermining that joint work should necessarily be concerned with human rights, democracy or pluralism (though schools quite often choose to do this); it is rather that the structured use of ICT facilitates collaborative work, and the process of working together on a joint enterprise opens up opportunities for respecting difference and celebrating diversity. Debate about the nature of citizenship, at least in Northern Ireland, has so far largely ignored the place of 'virtual contact' through ICT and its proven capacity to generate discourse. Evidence from the work carried out since 1986 outlined in this chapter shows that ICT, when it is effectively managed, can help to build trust. And trust makes it possible for participants to share ideas about those issues that divide them as well as those that unite them. In short, we assert that if ICT is considered only as a tool for improving academic learning it misses the massive potential for enriching human values and developing social capital.

Second, work of this nature will only become embedded in schools when sufficient account is taken of two very significant conceptual issues. The first relates to teachers. Considerable work has been done in Northern Ireland and elsewhere in defining what is meant by teacher 'competence':[5] much of this relates to the ability to manage learning effectively in the classroom but relatively little weight has been attached to what has been called 'intercultural competence' (Davis et al., 2005). Davis argues that intercultural competence 'can be defined as transformation of learning and a growth process where an individual's existing, often implicit, knowledge is diversified to intercultural knowledge, attitude, and behavior. The learning and growth process allows individuals to incorporate intercultural knowledge into their high level cognitive schema'.

She quotes Leeman and Ledoux (2003) to make the case that such competency should not be an extra facet of teachers' professional development but an integral part of it. While the General Teaching Council for Northern Ireland has adopted a set of professional values for teachers, this does not include anything as specific as intercultural competence. To enable teachers and the guardians of professional standards to engage in discussion about this role in education, a second conceptual issue will need to be addressed.

This is concerned with how schools define themselves and their function in society; following the pioneering work of Istance (2004a; 2004b) and McCluskey (2004), schools are being invited to imagine what 're-schooling' might look like, with schools as 'learning organisations' making extensive use of ICT to connect the school as an institution to the local and global community. This vision is a long way from the school as an organisation devoted to the transmission of knowledge or simply preparing young people to succeed in examinations. Falling rolls in post-primary schools in Northern Ireland offer a particularly interesting opportunity for policy-makers and teachers to consider how the educational ICT infrastructure can be used to support joint work between schools in the delivery of the new broader academic and vocational curriculum and in so doing, reconnect young people. Making such a paradigm shift in educational thinking will not be easy, but it will equip young people with the digital literacy skills they need to survive in an inter-dependent global society. This position would be cost-effective, would embed high-level ICT skills in the emerging work force and would make an important contribution to social cohesion within Northern Ireland.

Notes

1   Elections in March 2007 have resulted in the possibility of devolved administration in Northern Ireland at the time of writing.
2   The Women's Coalition decided to disband in 2006.
3   Austin, R. (1992) A European dimension in the curriculum: the role of satellite TV and electronic mail. *Learning Resources Journal*, 8(1), February, 8–13.
      Austin, R.(1992) European studies through video-conferencing. *Learning Resources Journal*, 8(2), 1992, 28–31.
      Austin, R. (1992) A new view of Ireland, Britain and Europe. *Head Teachers Review*, Winter, 6–8.
      See also http://www.european-studies.org/ (accessed 1 May 2006).
4   www.dissolvingboundaries.org.
5   General Teaching Council for Northern Ireland, Code of Values and Professional Practice, www.gtcni.org.uk (accessed 7 May 2006).

11 Chattering classes

The moderation of deliberative forums in citizenship education

Ross Ferguson

The wake of any general election should be a time of optimism as Parliament gets a fresh start, fresh faces and potentially fresh impetus. However, the mood around Westminster following the two most recent general elections has been somewhat marred by successive low turnouts. As Philip Gould, Labour's polling guru, describes, it is as if politics is a game being played out in front of increasingly empty stadiums (Gould, 2003). Although analysis of the data reveals this trend has been underway for some time, the 2001 general election was a watershed. Turnout dropped to its lowest point since 1918, with fewer than 60 per cent of eligible voters showing up at the ballot box. Four years later, in 2005, and despite a major effort by the political class to encourage participation, just 61 per cent cast a vote.

Such figures have depressed many and alarmed others, with some commentators warning of a 'crisis of democracy'. While such claims may be slightly exaggerated, there is no doubt that a significant proportion of the British public has become disconnected from formal politics. What should concern us most is who those people are. For it is beneath the superficial, headline statistics that the real cause for alarm may be found. While turnout may be down among the population in general, it is at its lowest among the youngest voters, with fewer than 40 per cent of 18- to 24-year-olds making their mark in 2001. Whilst the general turnout was up in 2005, among the 18–24s it fell further, to 37 per cent.

The '2001 experience' served as a catalyst for two principal debates about political engagement that remained current in 2006: what can be done to get young electors back into the 'stadium' at polling time, and what can be done to bring them off the political sidelines in the period between elections? Among the proposed solutions, the favourite was the introduction of citizenship education into the national curriculum. Momentum was provided by the Crick Report, which demonstrated that political engagement during childhood positively impacted on awareness and participation once the age of electoral majority had been reached (QCA, 1998).

Citizenship was made a statutory requirement in the English curriculum in 2002 (with non-statutory variations appearing in the curricula of the other home nations). Political literacy is just one of the three 'strands' making up citizenship education; tellingly, both Ofsted and NFER (in its excellent longitudinal study) have reported it is also the weakest and hardest to deliver (Clever *et al.*, 2005; DfES, 2005).

Many of those delivering citizenship education in schools regard the political literacy strand as under-resourced, unfamiliar and, as a result, a potentially frustrating part of their teaching duties. Anecdotal evidence from students also attests to the unease with which they approach citizenship. After all, 'politics' as it conventionally appears in mainstream media is as remote from the lives of young people as pension schemes (and certainly no more exciting). The NFER's observations in schools reveal that the learning environment for political literacy continues to be based in the classroom using traditional teaching methods involving working from a textbook and listening to the teacher, with few opportunities given over to discussion and debate.

To help address some of the deficiencies outlined above, and make citizenship education engaging and interesting to both those who learn and teach it, the Hansard Society launched the *HeadsUp* website (www.headsup. org.uk) in 2003. *HeadsUp* is an experiment to investigate how information and communication technology (ICT) can be utilised to aid learning and teaching experiences. As the site has developed we have seen that ICT can create a platform where learning can be taken beyond the classroom, where complex subjects can be made more accessible and where learning about politics can be achieved through 'doing' politics. This chapter provides a practitioner's account of how the use of 'online moderation' has proved integral to the success of the early development *HeadsUp*.

Doing politics

In May 2006, there were over 270 schools registered on *HeadsUp*, with around 3,260 individual students signed up. *HeadsUp* is about providing a place where young people under the age of electoral majority, parliamentarians and teachers can come together to engage with political events, issues and policies. It is the 'doing politics' that has made *HeadsUp* popular among young people and helped them to develop the skills that can sustain their contributions to the political process. For teachers it is an opportunity to deliver an interactive, productive lesson, and for politicians it is a rare opportunity to get into structured dialogue with Britain's young citizens.

The centrepiece of the site is its deliberative forum. While interaction between young people and mainstream political structures – such as voting and political parties – has declined, research and testimony reveal that their interest in activist and issue-based politics remains vibrant (Electoral Commission, 2002). All the topics for debate in the forum are suggested by the young people themselves. Seventeen debates have been held since the site was launched – these have included immigration, anti-social behaviour, poverty and the 2005 general election. The key to *HeadsUp* is that these debates are timed to coincide with relevant parliamentary events, consultations and inquiries. Parliamentarians are then invited to join the debates and use the experience to inform their scrutiny and legislative work.

HeadsUp's direct impact on policy-making and scrutiny may be modest, but it is tangible. The voting and candidacy age forum was supported by the Electoral Commission, which was seeking evidence directly from young people for its 2003 inquiry into reform of the age of electoral majority. It was a noteworthy forum for young people's expressions of interest and respect for the electoral process and not their alienation from it. The young people's contributions to the forum were quoted extensively throughout the Electoral Commission's report, 'Age of Electoral Majority', published in April 2004.

With the Children's Commissioner debate in September 2004, parliamentarians directly consulted with young people on proposals for a children's commissioner. Findings from the forum were referenced by MPs on the floor of the Commons during debate of the bill, and the DfES included the forum contributions in the application material sent to candidates for the commissioner position that was eventually created. As the site has increased in visibility and young people have shown themselves to be very capable of dealing with complex issues and discussing them, so politicians have been more confident and enthusiastic about getting involved. Debates held in 2006 involved an average of seven elected representatives per forum drawn from across the political spectrum. *HeadsUp* users, parliamentarians and schools welcomed the forums during the build-up, event and aftermath of the general election and G8 summit in 2005, as a route through which young people could contribute to the public debate and excitement around major political affairs. The G8 debate greatly benefited from the dialogue between the young people and MPs from across the political spectrum, including the Minister for International Development – who pursued the opportunity while on a fact-finding mission in Sudan. After the close of the forum, the minister wrote to the participants drawing attention to the parallels between the conclusions of the forum and the discussions at the summit itself.

Importance of moderation

Most forms of offline deliberation employ chairing or refereeing techniques to preserve their structure and deliver on objectives. Interactive online platforms, such as mailing lists and chat rooms, also have some form of administration or editing in place. The equivalent of chairing in an online deliberative forum is 'moderation' (sometimes also known as 'eModeration'). However, despite being similar in spirit, moderation differs in some very fundamental aspects to its offline equivalents. Whereas chairing takes place in 'real time' within set physical parameters, the nature of the online medium makes interaction between participants and moderation almost entirely asynchronous and incorporeal.

The necessity for moderation in deliberative online forums is what distinguishes these exercises from chat rooms, bulletin boards or email groups. Stephen Coleman and John Gotze described discussions that took place on the latter platforms as 'free-for-alls' that require: 'no rules or regulation, no attempt to reach a conclusion, no summary of what is said and no feedback. In free-for-all discussions anyone can say anything, but no one can have much expectation of being heard or influencing policy outcomes' (Coleman and Gotze, 2001: 16). Moderation, then, is integral to making online deliberation worth participating in, from the point of view of citizens, and worth running in relation to the cost, time and quality-concerns of Parliament, government, political parties or elected representatives.

Online deliberations vary in their purpose and thus require different types of participants, time frames and resource material. They also require different moderation strategies depending on the stage a deliberation is at and the dynamics at work between the participants (White, 2006). *HeadsUp* employs the same strategies used in any deliberative forum. However, rather than delivering moderation through a single detached moderator, in the case of *HeadsUp* a cast of characters were devised, each with its own role to play. These characters are adopted by trained and security-vetted staff from the Hansard Society's Citizenship Education Programme, who are then able to moderate from within the flow of the forums alongside the participants.

Hosting deliberation

When a forum opens, the first duties of a moderator are that of the 'host'. During the lifetime of a forum a community (or network) of participants is created. The people who constitute 'the community' will all start as strangers to one another; indeed, they are likely to remain that way. This can be especially true of *HeadsUp* where the student participants are anonymous and can be separated by significant distances and differences in socioeconomic background.

On *HeadsUp*, the host of the forums is 'MasterZen'. This character has an appearance similar to that of an elderly but jovial Shaolin monk. The design of this character references wry philosophical characters from movies and television programmes (for example, the 'Yoda' character in the *Star Wars* franchise). 'MasterZen' is used to open and close every forum; over the duration, his character is objective, never takes a particular side in a debate and is always friendly with every participant.

Moderators perform this 'host' role to ensure that the deliberation space retains an atmosphere conducive to expression and exchange of ideas and views. The 'host-moderator' can make participants feel welcome, ensure everyone has the information they need to take part, that they feel positive about participation in the forum and that they are aware of the context within which the deliberation is taking place. As the discussions progress, moderators can make sure that the momentum and participant interest are sustained. This can include bringing 'splinter' groups back into the main discussion, bringing new arrivals up to speed or introducing new pieces of information for consideration (references to TV programmes or video games, for example).

HeadsUp forums are often held to feed directly into consultations or parliamentary inquiries, and so the achievement of specific objectives is dependent on keeping within time constraints. Moderators have an important managerial role to play in this respect. In the planning stages of a consultation, timetables should be constructed and critical points identified (such as the close of deliberation within a certain topic-space or the airing of a relevant television programme). Over the course of the forum, moderators pay close attention to the schedule and are responsible for introducing reminders into the flow of the debate for the benefit of participants.

Dealing with conflict

In addition to clear timetables, good forums require defined rules and etiquette – some of which are familiar across community sites online, while others are specific to a particular site. *HeadsUp* participants are required to formally acknowledge the site's terms and conditions during registration. These include reminders about safety online and keeping contributions focused on the topic in hand.

Disagreement is an inevitable – and welcome – part of a deliberative process (Sunstein, 2003). However, participants who are inexperienced in debating, or less informed about the specific subject matter, may find this facet of participation uncomfortable and off-putting. At the other extreme, there may be those who 'spoil for an argument' or are so convinced by the faultlessness of their argument that they overreact to disagreement.

Dealing with conflict is one of the more testing and consequential roles of the moderator. In the vast majority of *HeadsUp* forums, participants avoided direct contention, chose their words carefully, used evidence to back up a point or were happy to accommodate different perspectives simultaneously. In this respect, participants were self-moderating and even on occasion self-policing, in that where disagreement occurred between individuals other participants stepped in to remind them of the rules, requested supporting evidence, asked for clarification or insisted on restraint. Such 'participant-to-participant' moderation is informally encouraged but it remains the policy on *HeadsUp* for the moderators to have the overall authority and responsibility for resolving conflict.

Moderators in their 'referee' role are there to reassure participants. They exist so that participants know that as long as they stay within the general rules and context of the topic, they are able to say what they want without fear. They also know that they are able to challenge contributions that they believe are wrong, in need of further qualification or could be superseded. Online consultations can be kept secure, structured but unconstrained, and the only way that this can be sustained is if the citizens and parliamentarian participants both have trust in the moderators to be decisive, fair and neutral.

Where *HeadsUp* moderators have to step in to resolve conflict then they must do so in a determined manner. This form of moderation is delivered through three characters. The main character in upholding the rules is 'Justice' who, while wearing the clothes of a legal professional also has a hint of tasteful glamour about her. Justice is joined by her deputies the laid-back hipster, 'Chilli', and the less-than-sunny, 'Gruff'. 'Chilli' and 'Gruff' are often brought into play before 'Justice' to suggest other points of view (positive and negative, respectively) in bids to quell or distract prickly, stagnating arguments.

Disputes are rarely between camps and more often between individuals. If and when participants get into a disagreement, some time is given to allow self-resolution. If a settlement is not reached, moderators aim to resolve the matter in public in the forum space. It is the aim of this approach to show the participants how to deal with the conflict themselves. On rare occasions, moderators will decide to suspend participant accounts until the individual(s) either express a lack of interest in continuing or pledge to change tack. Indefinite blocking of a participant has yet to happen – if such a move is necessitated all the participant details and a record of contributions remain stored on the site. In each case where off-forum action is required, the moderation team take their lead from the student's teacher as to whether and when to reinstate their access to the forum.

'Refereeing' is a big responsibility for moderators – it requires training and experience but also the ability to consult with other moderators and teachers. Yet again, it is important to stress that incidences of serious, irresolvable disagreement or rule-breaking in general have happened rarely in the life of *HeadsUp* or the Hansard Society's wider experience of online deliberation. This is due to having moderation planned in at an early stage, a clear statement of moderator responsibilities, visible moderator presence and a set of terms and conditions for participants, which they pledge to honour.

Promoting informed discussion

HeadsUp's moderators are required to have a good level of awareness around a forum's subject matter. The rationale behind this is not just so that moderators are able identify instances where participants are misusing or purposefully omitting information; it is also vital because the young people often seek information directly from the moderators or more specifically from the site's sassy intellectual, 'BigEd'.

The moderators do not need to wait for students to ask for information or make mistakes. Part of 'Big Ed's' role is to encourage use of evidence, facts and figures by participants and to signpost useful information. Bringing new information into discussions or referencing interesting sources has proved to be an excellent way to reinvigorate a discussion and encourage creative thought on the part of the students, which in turn provides parliamentarians with a richer seam of evidence.

The moderator's 'librarian' intervention is reinforced by a set of rudimentary background notes that may, for example, explain the content of a bill, outline the responsibilities of a select committee or provide a glossary explaining topic-related jargon. This background material is compiled and written up specifically for young people by the moderators. Teachers are able to use this reference material alongside the lesson plans provided to help teachers prepare their students before the forum opens. The students are also encouraged to cite the information in their posts alongside that which they research for themselves.

Moderation by teachers and parliamentarians

The moderation on *HeadsUp* provides both a partnership and a support mechanism for citizenship education teachers. The degree of moderation per class is dependent on the extent of pre-forum preparation carried out by teachers. Where teachers have gone through the lesson plans, allowed their students time to peruse the background information and spent time discussing issues with their classes beforehand, the amount of intervention from the Hansard Society's moderators decreases. Students who are underprepared call on the moderators more frequently, and give more reason for the moderators to interject in the interaction between participants.

Teachers can, of course, provide a distinct 'moderation' role of their own. During *HeadsUp*'s first year, the Hansard Society spent a lot of time visiting schools to observe the use of the site by teachers as a classroom resource. As a result of those observations, the focus on the teachers' role was shifted away from simply preparing students to encouraging them to actively discuss the topics and contributions with their students while they were logged on to the site. This may seem an obvious way for teachers to direct their involvement whilst their class is logged-on, but as the NFER study has demonstrated, debate and group activity has been all too rare in citizenship lessons.

The presence of parliamentarians in the forum also reduces the need for facilitation by the site's moderators. The purpose of *HeadsUp* is to provide a platform for dialogue between young people and their elected representatives, and when both parties engage in debate the moderators are eager to step aside and let either the parliamentarians or the students take the lead in setting the agenda.

The opportunity to get into debates with MPs has proved to be the principal incentive for young people using of the site. The best dialogues on *HeadsUp* have been those where the parliamentarians tap into this enthusiasm and use the opportunity to properly engage the students in detailed conversations about policies, compromises and constructive solutions via a medium that affords the young people the space and time to consider and respond in their own voice. In short, where parliamentarians take on the facilitation role of the moderators the *HeadsUp* 'experience' is stronger for all involved. Of course, good moderators know when to step in and out of the dialogue, which is a skill that can only be picked up through participation in these forms of deliberation and by remaining responsive to feedback from participants.

Future development

This chapter has discussed moderation in the context of online deliberative consultations, with specific reference to *HeadsUp* and its use in the classroom. However, the example is instructive when considering other forms of ICT-led deliberation for use in other contexts. Parliament is one such context where ICT promises to play an increasingly prominent role in facilitating a new kind of democratic dialogue.

Parliament's use of online media for deliberative consultation is less than a decade old and not yet mainstreamed. As the usage of online deliberative consultations escalates, so moderation will mature as a practice. As participants – public and parliamentarian – become more familiar and competent with the technology, dynamics and scope, perhaps moderation will be reconfigured. There may be the opportunity for moderation to become an automated process, or a responsibility shared between participants. However, there will always be a case for at least the coordination of moderators by an expert body, particularly where politics, Parliament, government, policy and conflicting interests are concerned.

Whichever form it eventually takes and whichever strategies are employed, moderation should be non-partisan, transparent and rigorously applied. Moderators must work independently for both those consulting and those being consulted, and they must be trusted in equal measure by both groups. If this is achieved then the online deliberation process will be robust and revealing, with the potential to gather evidence efficiently and effectively as a supplement – if not an alternative – to conventional consultation methods.

12 How democracies have disengaged from young people

Stephen Coleman

In this chapter I argue that it is not young people that have disengaged from politics, as critics commonly lament, but contemporary political culture that has become disconnected from the language, values and aspirations of young people. In a world of interactive communication, politics still takes the form of a one-way conversation which is remote from daily experience, over complicated, demographically exclusive, excessively solemn and unlikely to result in tangible consequences.

According to an ICM survey of 16- to 20-year-olds, conducted for the Electoral Commission, 90 per cent say that they have no involvement in politics, but 60 per cent say that they would like to have more say in the running of the country (Hansard Society/Electoral Commission, 2004). There is clearly a connection to be made between democratic aspiration and active participation. When asked about their attitudes to politics, young people are eager to express their feelings of abandonment by the political system:

> If they're not going to listen to us, why should we listen to them?
> > (15-year-old girl from a teenage pregnancy unit, quoted in Review of the UK Youth Parliament, DfES, May 2004)

> There is a general feeling between politicians and the general public that it's a kind of them and us situation. There is them who are making the decisions and us who don't get their opinions heard.
> > (Young person, quoted in Henn *et al.*, 'A Generation Apart? Youth a Political Participation in Britain Today', *The British Journal of Politics and International Relations*, 4(2), 167–92)

Rather than concentrate upon the narrow normative conceptions of the political that have traditionally characterised pedagogies and campaigns directed towards the encouragement of 'active citizenship', my aim in this chapter is to explore emerging participatory models shaped around aspects of popular culture. The interaction of millions of young people with the reality TV show, *Big Brother,* provides a focus for this exploration.

Seeking clues in popular culture: *Big Brother* viewers and the 2005 British general election

Big Brother viewers and voters are predominantly young and female (Hill, 2002; Jones, 2003; Coleman, 2003). The success of *Big Brother*'s interactive relationship with its mass audience raises stimulating questions about the scope for mediating political relationships along similar lines. The idea of broadening the scope of the political to incorporate themes and emphases more commonly associated with popular culture resonates with a growing sense within political-communication studies that the border between serious, rational, high politics and frivolous, distracting, low culture is less robust and significant than it once seemed to be (Brants, 1999). Delli Carpini and Williams have observed that:

> Politics is built upon deep-seated cultural values and beliefs that are imbedded in the seemingly nonpolitical aspects of public and private life. Entertainment media often provide factual information, stimulate social and political debate, and critique government, while public affairs media are all too often diversionary, contextless, and politically irrelevant.
>
> (Delli Carpini and Williams, 2001:161)

In a similar vein, Corner and Pels argue that 'official' politics has been catching up, blurring the boundaries and levelling the hierarchy between 'high' political representation and 'low' popular entertainment' (Corner and Pels, 2003: 2). The success of *Big Brother* in generating the kind of participatory enthusiasm among its interactive audience that most politicians would love to engender among the people they claim to represent ought not to be read as evidence of a terminal political malaise. On the contrary, the convergence of popular and political communicative styles could have an invigorating effect upon democracy, releasing civic energies that have atrophied over the long years of separation.

On the face of it, comparing ways in which politicians seek popular mandates to represent the public with ways in which *Big Brother* 'house-mates' act out their claims to be 'good guys' before voting audiences might seem to be absurd. Beyond the surface, however, both strategies entail performative appeals which are remarkably similar. Both rely upon similar claims to be authentic, sincere and consistent – and both, implicitly or explicitly, challenge onlookers to discover chinks in their moral armour; both are dependent upon voluntary, mass participation; both are compelled to adopt opportunistic stances intended to promote chances of winning and avoid losing. Both, indeed, are locked into a game, *Big Brother* explicitly so; politics popularly derided as such. The differences between these two approaches to representing the public are significant, not in demonstrating their distinct and incomparable nature, but in exploring how one succeeds in stimulating participatory energies which the other seems unable to reach.

Research design

The research reported here was designed to explore how *Big Brother* viewers and voters experienced the 2005 UK general election. It was clear from the outset that simply conducting a post-election survey asking them what they had done during the election campaign and what they had made of it would have been methodologically inadequate. Asking people to recall a month-long event, which might not have meant very much to them even as they were experiencing it, would be less useful than establishing a panel that could be monitored every few days with a view to collecting experiential and attitudinal data in a dynamic fashion. It was decided, therefore, to recruit a panel of 200 *Big Brother* viewers and voters who would be paid a small sum to complete regular surveys from the beginning of the campaign until shortly after polling day. The panel was recruited by YouGov from a representative sample poll of people aged over 18. Ninety-three per cent of panel members responded to eight or more of the ten surveys.

Replicating the demography of the *Big Brother* audience, 75 per cent of panel members were female and 25 per cent male. Thirty-two per cent were aged between 18 and 25 and 37 per cent were aged between 25 and 31. Fewer than 2 per cent of panel members were aged over 39. All panel members described themselves as 'regular' viewers of *Big Brother* and 58 per cent of them stated that they had watched 'several hours' of the show each week during the 2004 series. This figure increased to 71 per cent for 25- to 39-year-old females, but fell to only 49 per cent for males in the same age group. Forty-seven per cent reported that they had voted in the 2004 series. Again, young women were much more likely to be *Big Brother* voters, with over half (56 per cent) of 25- to 39-year-old females having voted, compared with only 40 per cent of males of the same age. Most panel members who had voted in 2004 had cast their votes from home via landline telephones, but, interestingly, the majority of under 25s had cast their votes via SMS. Although multiple voting is allowed (indeed strongly encouraged) in *Big Brother,* three out of four voters stated that they cast just one vote in each eviction, while one in four reported casting the same vote up to five times. Fifty-six per cent of panel members and 82 per cent of panel members who had voted in the 2004 series reported that they had visited the official *Big Brother* website. Some 45 per cent of voters had visited the online discussion forum (females were twice as likely to have done so as males) and 7 per cent had posted messages in the forum. Three out of four (75 per cent) voters said that they had talked with other people about how they would vote before their votes were cast.

The close proximity of the European parliamentary election (in June 2004) and the 2004 series of *Big Brother* provided an interesting opportunity to explore whether *Big Brother* voters were more or less likely than others to cast a political vote. Asked whether they had voted in the European election (for which the national turnout was 38.2 per cent), only one in five reported that they had, falling to 12 per cent among 18- to 24-year-old females. As the graph below (Figure 12.1) shows, panel members who had voted in the 2004 series of *Big Brother* were significantly less likely to have voted in the European election than the average British citizen, even when age comparisons are taken into account.

The Prime Minister called the 2005 general election on 5 April and Parliament was dissolved on 11 April. Polling day was on 5 May. Ten surveys were conducted between 12 April and 10 May. Over one hundred survey questions were asked, intended to probe how panel members experienced the general election campaign. This was achieved by asking respondents detailed questions about their behaviour within the previous 24 hours, their recollection of political messages and their attitudes towards a range of issues, politicians and institutions.

Binary responses to survey questions are inherently limiting. In order to enable panel members to articulate in their own terms what it felt like for them to be citizens of a democracy during an election campaign, each of the ten surveys was concluded with an unfinished sentence which respondents were asked to complete in their own words. These sentences were designed to stimulate candid and unrehearsed comments from panel members. These qualitative responses, which amounted to 18,771 words, were then analysed with a view to deriving qualitative interpretations.

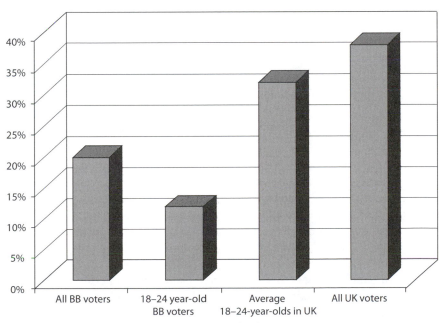

Figure 12.1 Voting in the 2004 European Election

Big Brother viewers as active citizens

The relaxed and obligation-free relationships that the audience has with *Big Brother*, as entertained viewers, discriminating judges, interactive participants and empowered voters, signals a new kind of citizenship which combines the autonomy and flexibility of the audience with the collective decision-making of the traditional political public. One might characterise this hybrid as remote-control citizenship. Although democratic theorists have tended to be understandably uneasy about what Bernard Manin has called 'audience democracy' (Manin, 1997), regarding it as a slippery slope to populism, there are grounds for thinking more positively about the convergence between contemporary audiences and publics. (Livingstone, 2005). As social reality has become increasingly a matter of mediated experience, one might reasonably argue that publics and audiences are essentially the same people going through the same process of trying to make sense of a world that can only ever be apprehended indirectly. Indeed, as we have suggested, active, critical audiences may well be more discriminating in their sense-making than publics driven by blind duty or deaf indifference. If, as most democratic theorists now accept, the will of the public is best formed and expressed within the context of a public sphere where 'private people come together as a public' (Habermas, 1989), then the mass media and their increasingly interactive audiences are the closest we have at the moment to such a space for public reflection. The kind of debates about public tastes in architecture, which surrounded the BBC's *Restoration* series or about sexual identity, which resulted from the appearance of a transsexual on *Big Brother*, simply could not take place on the same scale in any other contemporary national space. It is in the mediated public sphere that publics and audiences converge to become remote-control citizens, free to switch off, switch channels, interact with media content and determine for themselves what matters to them and what does not.

The image of *Big Brother* viewers and voters as apathetic couch potatoes is not supported by the survey findings. Most of the panel members (51 per cent) described themselves as good citizens and more than one in three (38 per cent) claimed to be active citizens. But what did they mean by such self-descriptions – and by which criteria should we measure the validity of their claims? For this research, we selected three criteria which are sufficiently conventional to be recognised by political scientists who study participation, but sufficiently broad to capture wider elements of cultural citizenship. During the course of the 2005 election campaign, three aspects of panel members' behaviour were examined: gathering information about the election; talking to other people about the election and voting on election day.

Information gathering

Panel members were most inclined to trust television as their source of election information, with 58 per cent trusting television coverage of the election, compared to 12 per cent who trusted websites, 8 per cent who trusted newspapers and 3 per cent who trusted information received by word of mouth. Panel members placed twice as much trust in television correspondents (58 per cent) as in the parties' own manifestos and leaflets (24 per cent) to tell them what the parties stood for. Asked which sources they *least* trusted to tell them what the parties stood for, 47 per cent cited politicians' speeches and 46 per cent cited newspaper journalists.

Given that television was the most trusted medium, how much of the election campaign were panel members watching? More than one in five (22 per cent) said that they switched off the TV whenever the election was mentioned. This is actually lower than the national average during the 2005 campaign, in which, according to Ofcom research, 27 per cent of the population switched channels or switched off whenever election coverage came on, rising to 37 per cent among 18- to 24-year-olds (Ofcom, 2005: 23).

By the mid-way point of the campaign two-thirds (64 per cent) of panel members had seen a politician on TV, 48 per cent could specifically recall seeing the Liberal Democrat leader Charles Kennedy on their TV screens and 42 per cent recalled seeing some reference to the launch of the Conservative party manifesto. At the same mid-way point, fewer than one in four (23 per cent) stated that they had read an election leaflet, 9 per cent had watched Jeremy Paxman's interview with Tony Blair and not a single respondent had personally met a candidate. (The latter increased to a mere 2 per cent by the end of the campaign.) By the final week of the campaign, 71 per cent of panel members reported having seen Tony Blair on TV.

In the tenth survey, conducted shortly after polling day, 40 per cent of panel members reported that at some point during the campaign they had watched a party election broadcast (PEB) and 38 per cent had looked up information about the election online. These figures compare with 70 per cent of the UK population who claim to have watched a PEB (MORI, 5–10 May) and 15 per cent of the UK population who claimed to have used the Internet as a source of information about the election (Ward *et al.*, 2005). Thirteen per cent of panel members reported meeting a party canvasser during the course of the campaign, while UK citizens as a whole were twice as likely to have done so (MORI, 5–10 May). Some 0.5 per cent had attended an election meeting, a quarter of those who reported doing so in a nationally representative sample (MORI, 5–10 May).

It was in their use of new media that panel members seem to have been more active than the UK population as a whole. Even allowing for the fact that panel members all had Internet access (whereas only 60 per cent of the UK population did at this time), their use of the Internet in relation to the election campaign was significantly higher than Internet users as a whole. In Ward's survey of election related Internet use during the 2005 election campaign, 28 per cent of UK Internet users stated that they had gone online to seek information about the election and 5 per cent reported that they sent emails to others about the election. At the end of the first week of the campaign 10 per cent of panel members said that they had sent or received an email relating to the election within the past 48 hours and 40 per cent claimed to have visited a news website. Asked in the second week of the campaign about subjects raised in emails they had received over the past 48 hours, 34 per cent had received emails about romantic relationships, 26 per cent about money worries, 24 per cent about football, 10 per cent about TV soaps, 14 per cent about their local communities and 17 per cent about the election. In the final week of the campaign 10 per cent of panel members stated that they had visited a party website and 25 per cent had visited the BBC news website to find out more about the election.

Three days after the election, panel members were asked whether they had engaged in a number of different activities during the course of the campaign. Seventeen per cent had received an email from a friend about the election, 13 per cent had sent an email to a friend about the election and 38 per cent had looked up information about the election online. These findings suggest that *Big Brother* viewers were more likely to express themselves as active citizens in an interactive, online environment than in more traditional spaces of civic engagement. When this hypothesis was probed further, however, panel members seemed to regard the Internet as either an escape from the election or as a resource for gaining access to information in ways not available from the old media. Asked to complete the sentence, 'I have used the Internet during election campaign to . . .', approximately half of the respondents suggested that they went online in order to retreat from the election, stating that they used the Internet to 'access my Internet account and browse the web as normal – not to look at political campaign manifestos', 'avoid the election which is dominating the other media', 'get some news other than elections' or 'shop, surf and ignore the election'. Others used the Internet to 'make sure I'm making the right decision', 'do one of those quizzes to see which party I'm most aligned to' or 'try to work out where parties stand on certain issues, as it is not always clear from the sniping and evasion seen on TV'. In responses to several of the qualitative questions, enthusiasm was expressed for the opportunities presented by interactive media. Repeatedly, when asked how the general election could be made more accessible to them, panel members spoke of the need for 'more interaction between parties and the public on policy creation' and 'more interactive interviews with politicians'. It was not always clear how respondents imagined such an interactive relationship, but there was a clear sense that its absence somehow limited the effectiveness of contemporary political communication.

Talking about the election

There is a strong relationship between talking about politics and engaging in the democratic process. As McKuen argues, 'the act of public expression itself transforms subconscious sentiments into conscious cognition and provides the basis for an active rather than a passive political involvement' (McKuen, 1990). Some scholars argue that talking about civic issues constitutes political action in itself (Gamson, 1988) and most accept that interpersonal communication is a strong predictor of participatory behaviour (Horan, 1971: 650; Mutz, 2002; Weaver *et al.*, 1992).

Asked in the first week of the campaign, 60 per cent of panel members said that they had talked about the election with members of their family, 36 per cent with workmates, 29 per cent with a close friend and 4 per cent with a stranger. One in five (21 per cent) had not talked about the election with anyone. By the final week of the campaign, 64 per cent reported that they had had a conversation with someone else about how they would be voting, and almost a third (32 per cent) said that they had discussed the question of Tony Blair's honesty with someone else. Some 17 per cent had discussed the election with someone else via email.

Asking people whether they were 'talking about the election' reveals only part of the story, for some panel members were more interested in discussing other political issues which they considered more important than which party would form the next government of the UK. In the second week of the campaign panel members were asked what issues most concerned them. Just under half (44 per cent) said that they cared who won the election, while 60 per cent expressed concern about global warming, 40 per cent about the presence of British troops in Iraq and 32 per cent about the success of London's bid to host the 2012 Olympic Games (Figure 12.2). In short, for some panel members other political issues were more important than the election campaign that was dominating news coverage.

Non-election preoccupations were conspicuous when panel members were asked, in the second week of the campaign, which topics they had discussed with anyone else within the previous 48 hours. 56 per cent had talked about recent events in a soap opera, 53 per cent about personal money worries, 52 per cent about football, 46 per cent about the election, 25 per cent about their local community and 17 per cent about the state of the environment. The election competed for conversational attention among a range of issues, and the distinction between political and non-political topics of conversation were not always obvious.

Voting

Voting is a key measure of active citizenship – the crucial one for political scientists who equate turnout with participation. A week before the election, most panel members expressed an intention to vote, although almost a

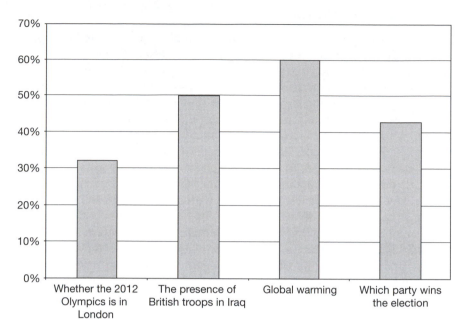

Figure 12.2 Which of the following are important to you?

third (31 per cent) were still unsure who they would vote for, and 12 per cent believed that they knew too little to cast a vote.

Almost two-thirds (64 per cent) of panel members regarded voting as a duty and a third (34 per cent) were in favour of compulsory voting. But when asked a few days before the election about factors which might prevent them from voting, 34 per cent stated that they were unable to decide who to vote for, 22 per cent expected to be too busy on election day and 19 per cent believed that their vote would make no difference (Figure 12.3).

In the post-election survey, 60 per cent of panel members claimed to have voted, 50 per cent at polling stations and 10 per cent by post. This was almost precisely the percentage of citizens who voted in the 2005 general election and higher than the average for the demographic group most represented on the panel. (Only 39 per cent of 18- to 25-year-olds voted nationally, but almost half (49 per cent) of panel members within the same age-group claimed to have voted.)

Big Brother viewers and voters were neither inattentive nor inactive citizens during the 2005 campaign. They did not sleep through the election, but their experience of the campaign was far from enthusiastic: 50 per cent of panel members stated that they found the campaign boring and 69 per cent said that they heard nothing during the course of the campaign that changed their minds about anything. Like most British citizens, they were

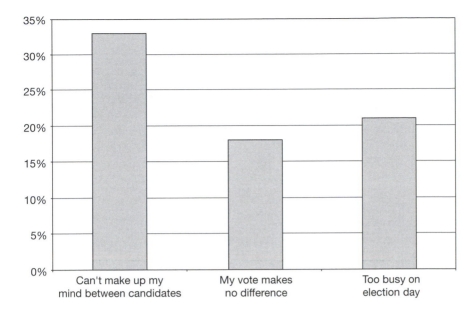

Figure 12.3 Which of the following would prevent you from voting?

reluctant participants in the election. The main reason for the sceptical and grudging nature of their participation was that they did not believe that their involvement in the election could have much impact on political consequences. In the language of political science, panel members had a very low level of political efficacy. (This concept refers to people's beliefs in their ability to understand and participate effectively in politics, as well as to their perception of the responsiveness of political institutions to their comments and demands.) Twenty-seven per cent believed that voting in the election would make no difference to the way the country is run; 37 per cent believed that politics was too confusing to follow; 41 per cent believed that nobody in government ever listens to them; 55 per cent said that anything they said or did would have no influence on how the country is run. Panel members' belief in their lack of influence reflected that of the national population; according to the British Election Study, 67 per cent of the UK population rated their influence on public affairs as between 0 and 3 out of 10, with 0 meaning no influence and 10 meaning much influence.

Low efficacy levels were linked to low expectations about the consequences of voting. Over half (53 per cent) of the panel members did not know the name of their elected MP three days after the election; 93 per cent did not expect to have any contact with their MP after the election, although one in four (25 per cent) expressed a wish to do so.

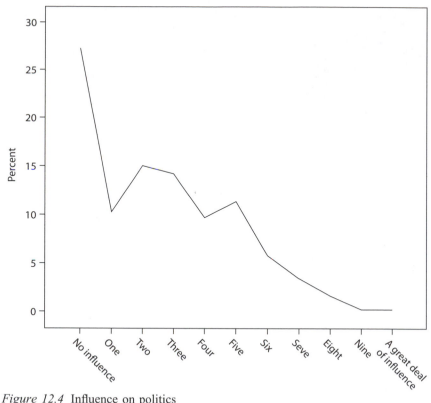

Figure 12.4 Influence on politics

Another perspective upon low efficacy was cast by the qualitative research. Asked in the first week of the campaign to complete the sentence, 'I'll only vote in the general election if . . .', over two thirds (69 per cent) of all responses expressed a lack of trust in the outcome of voting. Most panel members were only prepared to vote for a party or candidate if they felt confident that what was promised during the campaign would be delivered after the election. Typical completions of the sentence were '. . . if the parties involved show that they actually do what they state' and '. . . if I could be certain that the party I vote for would be true to themselves.' A second condition for voting, raised by approximately one in four of respondents, reflected anxieties about access to adequate information. For example, one respondent stated that they would only vote if 'I receive manifestos from each group in leaflet form, so at my own leisure I can read them and make an informed choice. (To date I have only received one leaflet!')

As remote control citizens, most panel members were more conscious of their remoteness from the political process than their control over it. They were faced with uncertainties about who or what could be trusted; access to balanced information; and whether their votes would lead to predictable outcomes. It was as if they had been repeatedly pressing the buttons on their remote controls, but there was nobody at the other end to receive their cries for assistance.

Representing authenticity

Both politicians and *Big Brother* candidates must appear before the cameras and perform. Performances require stages and staging. Symbolic settings matter (Edelman, 1985; Kertzer, 1988; Hajer, 2005). There is widespread contemporary distrust of staged appeals to the public: the mock sincerity of the eye-to-camera politician; the scripted eloquence of political speech-making; the chatty blog which was clearly written by an enthusiastic research assistant; the posed portraits of politicians and their stage extra families. From Major's humble soapbox to Blair and Cameron's abandonment of their once obligatory neckties, cultural democratisation requires would-be representatives to manifest ordinariness by appearing on the public stage as if they were offstage and being themselves. It is precisely this offstage lifeworld that the *Big Brother* format illuminates, providing its viewers with new ways to see and judge those who claim to speak for, or as the public. The drama of *Big Brother* is set within the private sphere of everyday intimacy. Although the show is but a mediated simulation of intimate life, its emphasis upon domestic interaction and shared experience conveys an impression of unrehearsed authenticity. Strategies usually associated with the traditional world of public politics, such as affected mannerisms, insincere claim-making and opportunist alliances, are precisely the forms of behaviour most likely to be punished by the onlooking public as they scrutinise the exposed domestic relationships of the *Big Brother* house.

Big Brother claims to depict real people dealing with everyday experiences: cooking and eating; gossiping and posing; sleeping and waking up; falling in love and having sex; getting drunk and suffering from hangovers; shopping and earning money; watching others and being seen; laughing and crying; winning and losing; arriving and leaving. It appeals to viewers' experience of the micro-political world of everyday relationships and mundane encounters with power. Viewers recognise such dramas from their own lives and are able to compare their own responses to those of the on-screen protagonists. *Big Brother* serves as a laboratory for the public observation of private conduct. In this sense, the political electorate and *Big Brother* voters are both engaged in the same game of judging the credibility of a group of distant others, only accessible to them via mediation. Hill argues that:

Reality gameshows have capitalised on [the] tension between appearance and reality by ensuring that viewers have to judge for themselves which of the contestants are being genuine. In fact, audiences enjoy debating the appearance and reality of ordinary people . . . The potential for gossip, opinion and conjecture is far greater when watching reality gameshows because this hybrid format openly invites viewers to decide not just who wins or loses, but who is true or false.

(Hill, 2002: 70)

Viewers of *Big Brother* are encouraged to adopt a paradoxical perspective towards the on-screen protagonists. On the one hand, they are outsiders looking in at an artificially-constructed private, domestic space in which 'ordinary people' are forced into intimate contact with one another. On the other hand, the house is manifestly a public space, constructed to be consumed by a mass audience, and the public's surveillant gaze is less an intrusion upon intimacy than a feature of participatory theatre. The project's success depends upon a constant and subtle tension between these private and public illusions. If the inmates of the house really believed that they were private and unobserved, their motivation to remain incarcerated would evaporate, but if they believed that they were constantly on show it would become impossible for them to maintain personal relationships. So, they live with ambiguity, experiencing both intimacy and exposure in much the way that one might when walking towards a CCTV camera in a shopping mall or posting to a chat room from one's bedroom or having a conversation on a mobile phone on a crowded bus.

Big Brother inmates deal with this ambiguous staging by imagining themselves to be in moments of either intimacy or exposure: the former in whispered conversations from one bed to another; the latter when dressing up and showing off for the Friday-night eviction show, as if suddenly they have consented to be seen by the outside world. Viewers also accept this ambiguity, sometimes seeing themselves as voyeuristic outsiders, and at others feeling like active participants in a public game.

In contrast, traditional political communication valorises the public over the private sphere, regarding the former as a space of shared rationality (Habermas, 1989), accountable visibility (Sennett, 1978) and collective solidarity (Putnam, 2000). In contrast, the private sphere is seen as atomised, feminised, emotive and inaccessible: a space of retreat from the civic and political world. Politicians have always had an uneasy relationship with personal intimacy and feel a need to patrol and control the border between private and public. Whereas talk for most people tends to be spontaneous and conversational, political speech (which often takes the form of speeches) is scripted and well-rehearsed, with off-the-cuff utterances regarded as risky paths to self-exposure. Whereas the subject of most people's talk is personal and experiential, politicians tend to speak impersonally and abstractly, steering the focus away from their own private lives.

But contemporary politicians are being dragged, sometimes kicking and screaming, into the sphere of mediated intimacy, undermining their well-crafted performances by exposing them to ever expanding public surveillance. Media-savvy politicians have responded by incorporating approved aspects of their private lives within their public performances, be it Tony Blair at the kitchen table with his children, George Bush taking a jog or Michael Portillo subjecting himself to the televised ordeal of pretending to be a single mother of four. In an age of mediated politics, the role of being a representative entails appearing to be someone who is extraordinary enough to represent others, but ordinary enough to be representative of others.

Whether they like it or not, political candidates are now judged in much the same way as *Big Brother* contestants. This means that they must accept the increased visibility of what was once strictly private and the need to invest emotionally in messages that could in the past have taken the form of impersonal publicity. As John Corner has astutely observed, politicians 'serve to condense "the political"' by embodying political values and ideas in ways that often exceed 'rationalistic commitments' (2000: 80). Just as *Big Brother* reflects a recognition that the personal is often political, contemporary obsessions with politicians' personas reflect an acknowledgement that the political is always bound to be personal, at least to the extent that one cannot credibly represent values without being seen to live them.

As the credibility of politicians is decreasingly determined by their ideological stances or partisan loyalties, and the judgement of volatile voters tends to revolve around questions of character integrity and witnessed reputation, the public stage of well-managed performance has a diminishing value. Politics is moving inside: spatially, to the observed private sphere in which duplicity cannot be sustained for long, and psychologically, towards an unprecedented public interest in the inner strengths, struggles and frailties of their leaders. Sennett regards this as a 'confusion' which 'has arisen between public and intimate life' and laments the fact that 'people are working out in terms of personal feelings public matters which properly can be dealt with only through codes of impersonal meaning' (Sennett, 1978: 5). But for many disengaged citizens, it is precisely the impersonal abstraction of most political talk that they find disingenuous and alienating. Clearly, there are aspects of discussion about complex social issues which are best conducted in the clinical terms of instrumental rationality, but need these be at the expense of subjective and affective perspectives which serve to connect grand policy-making to the democratic sensibilities of public experience?

Despite the tendency of political scientists to ignore the dramatic and affective aspects of political behaviour, preferring to see politics as an instrumentally driven competition between rational interests, there is much evidence to suggest that citizens' support for policies and politicians depends as much upon how they feel about them as what they know about them.

Politicians have always been judged on the basis of performative qualities, such as how convincingly they speak, whether they look like a leader, whether they appear calm under stress and whether they could be relied upon if they were a personal friend. Contrary to the rather condescending assumption that only the least educated and politically indifferent make judgements on such an affective basis, the opposite is in fact true: it is the better-educated, politically active citizens who are most likely to evaluate politicians on the basis of their personal qualities (Miller *et al.*, 1986). Because personality traits, ethical values and observable behaviour matter to citizens in making judgements about who is fit to represent them, the way in which these qualities are depicted is central to effective (and also affective) democracy.

When panel members were asked to complete the sentence, 'I would only support an election candidate if he or she . . .' the vast majority of respondents referred to notions of integrity and authenticity. The term 'genuine' was the most common epithet of approval. Typically, they stated that that they would only support a candidate who 'was down to earth and more real', 'shows humanity and admits weaknesses' or 'was approachable and naturally human'. It seemed from the qualitative research as if *Big Brother* voters wanted to judge political representatives in much the same way as they choose their own friends. They found politicians' claims to represent them too rhetorical, remote and non-transparent to be convincing. They wanted something else from representation: qualities and characteristics more universally human than the abstract promise-making of electioneering.

In the second week of the campaign, panel members were asked to state which two characteristics they would most want the candidate of their choice to possess. Most wanted their chosen candidate to be 'an ordinary person' (53 per cent) and 'a good listener' (52 per cent). The opposite characteristics were less popular: only 10 per cent wanted candidates to be extraordinary people and 23 per cent preferred them to be good talkers (Figure 12.5).

That was the ideal. When asked how, in reality, they would characterise the candidates standing in their constituency, only 17 per cent of panel members selected 'ordinary' and 9 per cent 'straight-talking', while 29 per cent chose 'slimey', 35 per cent 'arrogant' and 53 per cent 'false'.

Three days' before polling day, panel members were asked to select a number of qualities that would make a candidate appealing to them. Qualities rated least important included looking good on TV (1 per cent), knowing more than the voter (12 per cent) and having business experience (14 per cent). The most popular qualities were an ability to speak convincingly (49 per cent), having strong political values (40 per cent) and looking like an ordinary person (37 per cent).

When asked after the election to describe the characteristics of the MP elected in their constituency, most panel members were unable to state whether their elected representative was trustworthy (56 per cent), ordinary

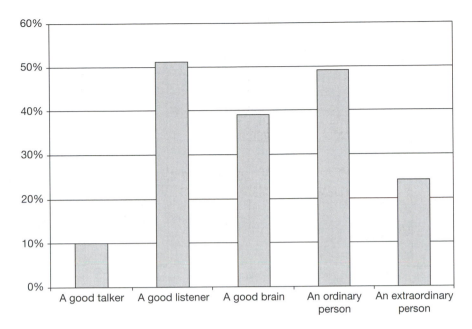

Figure 12.5 Which *two* of the following best describe the kind of politician that you would be likely to vote for?

(58 per cent), clever (59 per cent) or friendly (61 per cent). In short, a majority of panel members were unable to make informed judgements about the very characteristics that they considered to be most important in judging candidates.

Asked with whom they would most like to have a discussion about the state of the world, 39 per cent of panel members chose Tony Blair and 36 per cent selected Jamie Oliver. (These choices were well ahead of Jeremy Paxman and David Beckham, each at 10 per cent, and Michael Howard at 5 per cent). Asked shortly after the election which politicians and non-politicians would make good legislators, Jamie Oliver received more support (34 per cent) than Tony Blair (25 per cent), Jeremy Paxman (22 per cent) and George Galloway (2 per cent), but less than Bob Geldof (47 per cent).

Given the consistently strong support for Jamie Oliver as a credible political figure, panel members were asked to compare him with Tony Blair in terms of five characteristics (Figure 12.6). A significant majority of panel members felt that Oliver, more than Blair, has values, is 'real', gets things done and is like them. Jamie Oliver was even considered to make more difference to the world around him than Tony Blair!

The strong conclusion that emerges from these findings is that when *Big Brother* viewers and voters judge political leaders they reward similar

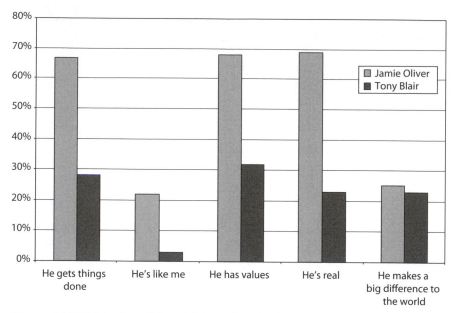

Figure 12.6 Think about Prime Minister Tony Blair and TV chef Jamie Oliver: which of the following statements applies to them?

characteristics to those which appeal to them as voters in *Big Brother*. They regard both contests as raising similar questions about the authenticity and ordinariness of people claiming to speak for and as the public. But panel members experienced considerable difficulty identifying these characteristics in political candidates; most were unable to draw any conclusions about qualities which they regarded as paramount in reaching a judgement about politicians, whereas they had no difficulty in determining these qualities in *Big Brother* housemates. These conclusions beg the question of whether an electoral system that was more like *Big Brother* – more emotionally accessible, permanently visible and directly interactive – would appeal to and engage *Big Brother* viewers and voters.

Asked whether they would rather vote in *Big Brother* or the general election, over one in four panel members chose the former, although a clear majority (69 per cent) placed greater value upon their political votes (Figure 12.7).

The panel was then asked whether they thought that the *Big Brother* format, in which candidates are under constant surveillance, with the least popular voted out each week, would be a better way of electing representatives than the present electoral system. A majority (54 per cent) did, although one in three (30 per cent) did not (Figure 12.8).

In an attempt to understand why a majority of panel members felt such confidence in their capacity to judge political candidates, they were invited

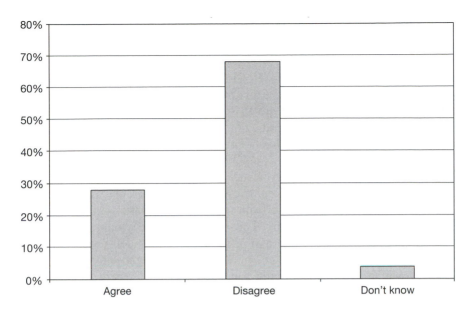

Figure 12.7 'I'd rather vote in Big Brother than the general election'

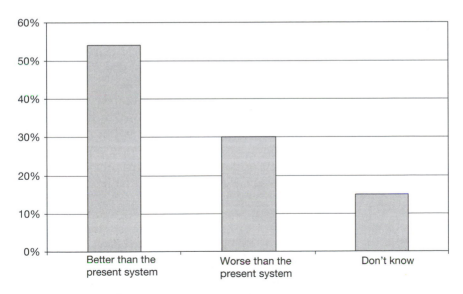

Figure 12.8 If the election were more like Big Brother, so that you could watch candidates in real-life situations and remove the one you least like, would this be . . .?

to complete the sentence, 'If *Big Brother* voters decided the result of the election, it would be better because . . .'. Respondents emphasised two different aspects of representation which they thought the *Big Brother* approach might enhance. First, they considered that representatives would be forced to become more exposed and open to emotional surveillance. In an election determined by *Big Brother* voters, they argued, 'We'd get to see the real person and we'd get to see a lot more of them', 'The most genuine person would win', and 'You may see the actual personality of the politician, not just the public person.' The result, they suggested, would be that 'the false candidates would be weeded out' and 'true character would be judged, rather than the facade'. Second, panel members considered that *Big Brother* voters would constitute a more representative electorate: 'You would get an overall vote from the entire population rather than the middle-class voters' view' and, 'The ordinary people would decide who represents them.' A clear impression given by respondents was that *Big Brother* voters could bring a degree of emotional intelligence to the electoral process, which is at present being squeezed out.

Reconnecting politics to the *Big Brother* generation

The image of *Big Brother* as a refuge for a politically distracted generation, squandering its precious votes on televised popularity polls while refusing to meet its civic obligations at the ballot box, reflects a hopelessly narrow conception of politics which assumes that the professionally devised agendas of political elites must be of greater value than those emanating from common experience. New orientations, aesthetics and languages of democratic participation are eroding the boundaries of the political, leading some to conclude that even the most sacred centrepiece of democratic architecture, the election campaign, is in need of cultural reinvention.

A key sense in which current political citizenship has become disconnected from the cultural citizenship of young people is manifested by the awkward-ness of most politicians, governments, parties and political journalists when faced with the new communicative demands of interactive digital media. Generally speaking, their response is to use digital media as forms of one-way broadcast transmission. Peter Bazalgette, the producer of *Big Brother,* argues that:

> For young people, involvement in . . . the media is now all about a conversation. It's a two-way process where they generate much of the material. Just look at *MySpace* or *Facebook* to see what I mean. The result is that young political activists of the future will need to be involved in a dialogue. I don't think our politicians have a clue about this wholly novel development.

The 'clue' that politicians miss is not simply a recognition of the affordances of digital technology, but an awareness that citizenship itself, as a cultural project, is no longer (if it ever was) rooted in the inert context of reception and consumption. Citizenship in an interactive media environment is best described, in the terms of Fairclough *et al.* (2006), as a 'communicative achievement', which gets 'away from preconceptions about what citizenship *is*, and looks at how it is *done* – at the range of ways in which people position themselves and others as citizens in participatory events'. This repositioning has three striking characteristics. First, it rejects the high civic decoupling of participation and pleasure, assuming that democratic self-representation and collective action are most authentic when embedded within the everyday rhythms and mundane experiences of young people themselves. Second, it does not shy away from affective encounters with power and broad cultural judgements about the performances of power-holders. Third, it respects informal, as well as formal, forms of discursive circulation. In short, it is not confined to the political spaces of conventional politics. It is creating new space, language, effects and affects. Appeals to young people to vacate these spaces and migrate to the dark caves of the political elite are bound to fall on deaf ears. If there is to be cultural migration, it is political democracy which must learn to engage with the next generation of sovereign citizens.

References

Aday, S. (2005) Why trust matters: declining political trust and the demise of American liberalism. *Public Opinion Quarterly, 69*(2), 330–2.

Allport, G.W. (1954) *The Nature of Prejudice*. New York: Addison-Wesley.

Althaus, S. and Tewksbury, D. (2000) Patterns of Internet and traditional news media use in a networked community. *Political Communication, 17*, 21–45.

Anderson, David A. and Cornfield, Michael (eds) (2003) *The Civic Web: Online Politics and Democratic Values*. Lanham, MD: Rowman & Littlefield.

Anderson, J. (2006) *Kore wan an desu ka*. Available at: www.ltscotland.org.uk/ ictineducation/connected/connected14/specialfeature/korewanandesuka.asp (accessed 7 May 2006).

Andolina, M. and Jenkins, K. (2004) 'Don't Write off the Kids Just Yet . . . Hopeful Prospects for Youth in the 2004 Election.' Paper presented at the Pre-APSA Conference on Political Communication. Chicago, IL, 1 September.

Andretta, M., della Porta, D., Mosca, L. and Reiter, H. (2002) *Global, Noglobal, Newglobal. La protesta di Genova contro il G8*. Rome: Laterza.

Arthur, J. and Davidson, J. (2000) Social literacy and citizenship in the school curriculum. *The Curriculum Journal, 11*(1), 9–23.

Audigier, F. (1998) *Basic Concepts and Core Competences of Education for Democratic Citizenship*. Strasbourg: Council of Europe.

Austin, R. (1992a) A European dimension in the curriculum: the role of satellite TV and electronic mail. *Learning Resources Journal, 8*(1), February, 8–13.

Austin, R. (1992b) European studies through video-conferencing. *Learning Resources Journal, 8*(2), June, 28–31.

Austin, R. (1992c) A new view of Ireland, Britain and Europe. *Head Teachers Review*, Winter, 6–8. See also: www.european-studies.org/ (accessed 1 May 2006).

Austin, R. (2004) History, ICT and values: a case study of Northern Ireland, in *Formacion de la Ciudadania: Las TICs y los nuevos problemas* (translated as Citizenship Training: ICTs and new problems), eds M. Munoz and D. Perez. Alicante, pp. 45–57.

Austin, R. (2006) The Role of ICT in bridge-building and social inclusion; theory, policy and practice issues. *European Journal of Teacher Education*, May.

Austin, R., Abbot, L. Mulkeen, A. and Metcalfe, N. (2003) Dissolving boundaries: cross-national co-operation through technology in education. *The Curriculum Journal, 14*(1), Spring.

Austin, R., Smyth, J., Mallon, M., Mulkeen, M. and Metcalfe, N. (2004) Dissolving boundaries. Supporting transformation in the classroom? Available at: www.dissolvingboundaries.org/ (accessed 30 May 2006).

Ayers, M.D. (2003) Searching for a collective identity in the feminist cyberactivist, in M. McCaughey and M.D. Ayers (eds), *Cyberactivism. Online Activism in Theory and Practice*. New York–London: Routledge, pp. 145–64.

Baddeley, S. (1997) Governmentality, in B. Loader (ed.), *The Governance of Cyberspace*. London: Routledge.

Baker, L., Wagner, T., Singer, S. and Bundorf, M. (2003) Use of the Internet and e-mail for health care information: Results from a national survey. *Journal of the American Medical Association, 289*, 2400–6.

Barber, M. (2001) *Teaching for Tomorrow in OECD. Observer*. Available at: www.oecdobserver.org/news/printpage.php/aid/420/Teaching_for-tomorrow.html.

Barlow, J.P. (1996a) *Thinking Locally, Acting Globally. Time*, 15 January. Online at: http://jcgi.pathfinder.com/time/magazine/article/0,9171,983964,00.html.

Barlow, J.P. (1996b) A Cyberspace Independence Declaration. *Cyber-Rights List*, 8 February. Online at: www.homes.eff.org/~barlow/Declaration-Final.html.

Barnett, C. (2003). *Culture and Democracy: Media, Space and Representation*. Edinburgh University Press.

Barney, D. (2004) *The Network Society*. Oxford: Polity.

Barr, T. (2002) The Internet and online communication, in S. Cunningham and G. Turner (eds) *The Media and Communications in Australia*. Sydney: Allen & Unwin, pp. 244–57.

Barraket, J. (2005) Online opportunities for civic engagement? An examination of Australian third sector organisations on the Internet. *Australian Journal of Emerging Technologies and Society, 3*(2), 17–30.

Bauer, M. and Gaskell, G. (2000) *Qualitative Researching with Text, Image and Sound: A Practical Handbook*. London: Sage.

Bauman, Z. (2005) *Liquid Life*. Cambridge: Polity.

Beck, U. (1998) *Democracy without Enemies*. Cambridge: Polity.

Beck, U. (2000) *What is Globalization?* Cambridge: Polity.

Bell, D. (2005) 'Education for Democratic Citizenship' speech for the Roscoe lecture series in Liverpool, 2 November. Available at: www.education.guardian.co.uk/ofsted/story/0,,1606888,00.html.

Bennett, L. (1998) The Uncivic Culture: Communication, Identity, and the Rise of Lifestyle Politics. *PS: Political Science and Politics, 31(4)*, 740–61.

Bentivegna, S. (2002) Politics and new media, in L. Lievrouw and S. Livingstone (eds), *The Handbook of New Media*. London: Sage, pp. 50–61.

Berelson, B. (1952) *Content Analysis in Communication Research*. Glencoe, IL: Free Press.

Bessant, J. (2000) Social action and the Internet: New forms of political space. *Just Policy, 19*(20), 108–18.

Bessant, J. (2004) Mixed messages: youth participation and democratic practice. *Australian Journal of Political Science, 39*(2), 387–404.

Bimber, B. (1998) The Internet and political transformation: populism, community, and accelerated pluralism. *Polity, 31*(1), 133–60.

Bimber, B. (2003) *Information and American Democracy: Technology in the Evolution of Political Power*. Cambridge, MA: Cambridge University Press.

Bimber, B. and Davis, R. (2003) *Campaigning Online: The Internet in U.S. Elections.* Oxford University Press.

Black, E. (1998) Digital democracy or politics on a microchip, in C. Alexander and L. Pal (eds), *Digital Democracy.* Oxford, Oxford University Press.

Bontempi, M. and Pocaterra, R. (eds) (2007) *I figli del disincanto. Giovanni e partecipazione politica in Europa.* Milano: Bruno Mondadori.

Brady, P.W., Thomson, L.F., Wuensch, K.L. and Grossnickle, W.F. (2003) Internet recruiting: the effects of Web page design features. *Social Science Computer Review*, 374–5.

Brants, K. (1999) Who's afraid of infotainment? *European Journal of Communication, 13*(3), 315–35.

Brown, G. (2006) We have renewed Britain; now we must champion it. *The Guardian*, 27 February, p. 32.

Bryman, A. (1998) Quantitative and qualitative research strategies in knowing the social world, in T. May and M. Williams (eds), *Knowing the Social World.* Buckingham: Open University Press, pp. 138–56.

Buckingham, D. (1999) Young people, politics and news media, *Oxford Review of Education, 25*(1–2), 171–84.

Buckingham, D. (2000) *After the Death of Childhood: Growing Up in the Age of Electronic Media.* Cambridge: Polity Press.

Cammaerts, B. and Van Audenhove, L. (2005) Online political debate, unbounded citizenship, and the problematic nature of a transnational public sphere. *Political Communication, 22*(2), 179–96.

Cammaerts, Bart and Carpentier, Nico (eds) (2006) *Reclaiming the Media: Communication Rights and Democratic Media Roles.* Bristol: Intellect Books.

Cairns, E. and Hewstone, M. (2001) *In Peace Education: The Concept, Principles and Practices Around the World.* Marwah, NJ: Larry Erlbaum Associates.

Carroll, B. (2004) *Culture Clash: Journalism and the Communal Ethos of the Blogosphere.* Online. Available at: www.blog.lib.umn.edu/blogosphere/culture_ clash_journalism_and_the_communal_ethos_of_the_blogosphere_pf.html (accessed 29 October 2004).

Cartocci, R. (2002) *Diventare grandi in tempi di cinismo.* Bologna: Il Mulino.

Cartocci, R. and Corbetta, P. (2001) Ventenni contro. *Il Mulino*, 5, 861–70.

Castells, M. (1996) *The Rise of the Network Society.* Malden, MA: Blackwell Publishers.

Castells, M. (1997) *The Information Age: Economy, Society and Culture. Vol. 2: The Power of Identity.* Oxford: Blackwell Publishers.

Castells, M. (2000) *The Rise of the Network Society.* Oxford: Blackwell.

Castells, M. (2001) *The Internet Galaxy. Reflections on the Internet, Business and Society.* Oxford: Oxford University Press.

Cavalli, L. and De Lillo, A. (eds) (1993) *Giovani anni novanta. Terzo rapporto Iard sulla condizione giovanile in Italia.* Bologna: Il Mulino.

CCEA (2003) Proposals for Curriculum and Assessment at Key Stage 3. Council for the Curriculum Examinations and Assessment. Available at: www.ccea.org.uk (accessed 14 May 2007).

Censis (2001) *XXXV Rapporto sulla situazione sociale del paese.* Milano: Franco Angeli.

Center For Media Education (2002) *TeenSites.Com – A Field Guide to the New Digital Landscape.* Washington DC: Center For Media Education (CME).

Chief Inspector's Report 2002–2004. Available at: www2.deni.gov.uk/inspection_ services/general_pub/Chief_Inspector_Report_02_04.pdf (accessed 31 May 2006).

Clark, L.S. (2005) The constant contact generation: exploring teen friendship networks online, in S. Mazzarella (ed.) *Girl Wide Web*. New York: Peter Lang, pp. 203–22.

Clever, E., Ireland, E., Kerr, D. and Lopes, J. (2005) Citizenship Education Longitudal Study: Second Cross-Sectional Survey 2004, QCA. London: QCA.

Cole, J., Suman, M., Schramm, P., Lunn, R. and Aquino, J. *et al.* (2003) The UCLA Internet Report: Surveying the Digital Future Year Three. UCLA Center for Communication Policy. Available at: www.digitalcenter.org/pdf/internetReport YearThree.pdf.

Coleman, J.C. (1993) Understanding adolescence today: a review. *Children and Society, 7*(2), 137–47.

Coleman, S. (2003) *A Tale of Two Houses: the House of Commons, the Big Brother house and the People at Home*. London: Hansard Society.

Coleman, S. (2005a) The lonely citizen: indirect representation in an age of networks. *Political Communication, 22*(2), 197–214.

Coleman, S. (2005b) *Remixing Citizenship*. London: Carnegie Young People Initiative.

Coleman, S. and Gotze, J. (2001) *Bowling Together: Online Public Engagement in Policy Deliberation*. London: Hansard Society.

Coleman, S. and Rowe, C. (2005) *Remixing Citizenship: Democracy and Young People's Use of the Internet*. London: Carnegie Young People Initiative.

Combs, J.E. and Nimmo, D. (1996) *The Comedy of Democracy*, Westport, CT: Praeger.

Corbetta, P. (1999) *Metodologia e tecniche della ricerca sociale*. Bologna: Il Mulino.

Corner, J. (2000) Mediated persona and political culture: dimensions of structures and process. *European Journal of Cultural Studies, 3*(3), 389–405.

Corner, J. and Pels, D. (eds) (2003) *Media and the Restyling of Politics*. London: Sage.

Cornolti, G., Cotti, F. and Bonomi, P. (2005) *WP8. Collection of Working Papers on National Survey Results. Italy – National Report*, EUYOUPART project.

Couldry, N., Livingstone, S. and Markham, T. (2006) *Media Consumption and the Future of Public Connection*. London: LSE Report, www.publicconnection.org.

Couldry, N., Livingstone, S. and Markham, T. (2007a). *Public Connection? Media Consumption and the Presumption of Public Attention*. Basingstoke: Palgrave Macmillan.

Couldry, N., Livingstone, S., and Markham, T. (2007b) Connection or disconnection? Tracking the mediated public sphere in everyday life, in R. Butsch (ed.), *Media and Public Spheres*. Basingstoke: Palgrave-Macmillan.

Crick, B. (1978) Basic concepts for political education, in B. Crick and A. Porter (eds), *Political Education and Political Literacy*. London: Longman.

Crick, B. (1998) *Education for Citizenship and the Teaching of Democracy in Schools*. London: QCA.

Crick, B. (2004) Why citizenship at all?', in B. Linsley and E. Rayment (eds), *Beyond the Classroom*. London: New Politics Network.

Crick Advisory Group (1998) *Education for Citizenship and the Teaching of Democracy in Schools*. London: QCA.

Cross, R. (1996) Geekgirl: why grrrls need modems, in Kathy Bail (ed.) *DIY Feminism*. Sydney: Allen & Unwin, pp. 77–86.

Cruikshank, B. (1999). *The Will to Empower: Democratic Citizens and Other Subjects.* Ithaca, NY: Cornell University Press.

Dahlgren, P. (2003) Reconfiguring civic culture in the new media milieu, in J. Curran and D. Pels (eds) *Media and the Restyling of Politics: Consumerism, Celebrity and Cynicism.* London: Sage.

Dahlgren, P. (2005) Internet, public spheres and political communication: dispersion and deliberation. *Political Communication, 22*(2), 147–62.

Dahlgren, P. (2006) Doing citizenship: the cultural origins of civic agency in the public sphere. *European Journal of Cultural Studies, 9*(3), 267–86.

Dahlgren, P. (2007) Civic identity and net activism: the frame of radical democracy, in L. Dahlberg and E. Siapera (eds) *Radical Democracy and the Internet.* London: Palgrave Macmillan.

Dahlgren, P. and Olsson, T. (2007) From public spheres to civic culture: young citizens' internet use, in Richard Butsch (ed.) *Media and Public Spheres.* Basingstoke: Palgrave-Macmillan, pp. 198–211.

Dahlgren, P. and Olsson, T. (2007) Facilitating political participation: young citizens, Internet and civic cultures, in S. Livingstone and K. Drotner (eds) *The International Handbook of Children, Media and Culture.* London: Sage.

Dalton, R.J. (2004) *Democratic Choices: The Erosion of Political Support in Advanced Industrial Democracies.* Oxford: Oxford University Press.

Davies, I. and Issitt, J. (2005) Reflections on citizenship education in Australia, Canada and England. *Comparative Education, 41*(4), 389–410.

Davies, I., Evans, M. and Reid A. (2005a) Globalising citizenship education? *British Journal of Educational Studies, 53*(1), 66–89.

Davies, I., Gorard, S. and McGuinn, N. (2005b) Citizenship education and character education. *British Journal of Educational Studies, 53*(3), 341–58.

Davies, L. (2006) Global citizenship. *Educational Review, 58*(1), 5–25.

Davis, N., Cho, M.O. and Hagenson, L. (2005) Intercultural competence and the role of technology in teacher education, in *Contemporary Issues in Technology and Teacher Education, 4*(4). Available at: www.citejournal.org/vol4/iss4/maintoc.cfm (accessed 7 May 2006).

de Jong, W., Shaw, M. and Stemmers, N. (eds) (2005) *Global Activism, Global Media.* London: Pluto Press.

della Porta, D. (1996) *Movimenti collettivi e sistema politico in Italia. 1960–1995.* Rome: Laterza.

della Porta, D. and Mosca, L. (2005) Global-net for global movements? A network of networks for a movement of movements. *Journal of Public Policy, 25*(1), 165–90.

della Porta, D., Andretta, M., Mosca and L., Reiter, H. (2006) *Globalization from Below. Transnational Activists and Protest Networks.* Minneapolis, MN: University of Minnesota Press.

Delli Carpini, M. and William, B. (2001) Let Us Infotain You: Politics in the New Media Environment, in W.L. Bennett and R. Entman (eds) *Mediated Politics. Communication in the Future of Democracy.* New York: Cambridge University Press, pp. 160–81.

Denegri-Knott, J. (2004) Sinking the online 'music pirates': Foucault, power and deviance on the web. *Journal of Computer-Mediated Communication, 9*(4). Available at: http://jcmc.indiana.edu/vol9/issue4/denegri_knott.html (accessed 14 May 2007).

DfEE (1999) *Citizenship Education Can Help Support Democracy.* Department for Education and Employment Press Release 276/99.

DfES (2005) *Listening to Young People: Citizenship Education in England.* Research Report 626. London: DfES.

Di Maggio, P., Hargittai, E., Neuman, R. and Robinson, J. (2001) Social implications of the Internet. *Annual Review of Sociology, 27,* 307–36.

Dixon, A. (2000) Fire blankets or depth charges: choices in education for citizenship. *Forum, 42*(3), 94–9.

Dordoy, A. and Mellor, M. (2001) Grassroots Environmental Movements: Mobilization in an Information Age, in F. Webster (ed.) *Culture and Politics in the Information Age.* New York and London: Routledge, pp. 167–82.

Dunleavy, P. (1996) Political behaviour: institutional and experiential approaches, in R. Goodin and H. Klingemann (eds) *A New Handbook of Political Science.* Oxford: Oxford University Press, pp. 276–93.

Dunleavy, P., Margetts, H., Bastow, S., Callaghan, R. and Yared, H. (2002) *Progress in Implementing E-government in Britain: Supporting Evidence for the National Audit Office Report.* London: The Stationery Office.

Dutton, W.H. (2005) 'Social Movement Shaping the Internet: The Outcome of an Ecology of Games'. Paper presented at the conference 'Extending the Contributions of Professor Rob Kling to the Analysis of Computerization Movements', The Berkman Center, UC Irvine, March.

Dwyer, P., Harwood, A. and Tyler, D. (1998) *Life-patterns, Choices, Careers: 1991–1998.* Melbourne: Youth Research Centre, Research Report 17.

Economist (2006) Who killed the newspaper? *The Economist,* 24 August.

Edelman, M. (1971) *Politics as Symbolic Action. Mass Arousal and Quiescence.* Chicago: Markham.

Edelman, M. (1985) *The Symbolic Uses of Politics.* Urbana, IL: University of Illinois Press.

ETI (2000) Report of a Survey of Provision for Education for Mutual Understanding in Post-primary School. London: ETI.

Electoral Commission (2002) *Voter Engagement and Young People.* London: The Electoral Commission.

Electoral Commission (2005) *Election 2005: Turnout. How Many, Who and Why?* London: The Electoral Commission.

Eliasoph, N. (1998) *Avoiding Politics: How Americans Produce Apathy in Everyday Life.* Cambridge: Cambridge University Press.

Enslin, P., Pendlebury, S. and Tjiattas, M. (2001) Deliberative democracy, diversity and the challenges of citizenship education. *Journal of Philosophy of Education, 35*(1), 115–30.

Ester, P. and Vinken, H. (2003) Debating civil society: on the fear for civic decline and the hope for the Internet alternative. *International Sociology, 18*(4), 659–80.

Eurobarometer (2000) *Measuring Information Society 2000,* 53 CEC, Brussels.

Eurostat (2005a) Internet activities in the European Union, in *Statistics in Focus,* 40.

Eurostat (2005b) 'Database', on-line. Available at: www.europa.eu.int/comm/eurostat (20 March 2005).

EUYOUPART (2005) *Political Participation of Young People in Europe,* on-line. Available at: www.sora.at/de/start.asp?b=14 (1 December 2006).

Evans, K. (2004) The significance of virtual communities. *Social Issues, 2*(1). Available at: www.whb.co.uk/socialissues/vol2ke.htm.

Fairclough, N., Pardoe, S. and Szerszynski, B. (2006) Critical discourse analysis and citizenship, in H. Hausendorf and A. Bora (eds) *Analyzing Citizenship Talk*. Amsterdam: John Benjamins, pp. 98–123.

Farrall, K.N. and Delli Carpini, M. X. (2004) 'Cyberspace, the Web Graph and Political Deliberation on the Internet.' Paper presented at the 2nd International Conference on Politics and Information Systems: Technologies and Applications, Orlando, Florida, USA, July.

Faulks, K. (2006) Education for citizenship in England's secondary schools. *Journal of Education Policy, 21*(1), 59–74.

Field, J. (2003) *Social Capital*. London: Routledge.

Foot, K.A. and Schneider, S.M. (2002) Online action in Campaign 2000: an exploratory analysis of the U.S. political web sphere. *Journal of Broadcasting and Electronic Media, 46*(2), June, 222–44.

Foot, K.A., Schneider, S.M. and Dougherty, M. (2005) 'Web Practices of Political Actors in the 2004 U.S. Congressional Election Web Sphere.' Presented at the International Communication Association Conference. New York, NY, 28 May.

Foot, K.A., Schneider, S.M., Kluver, R., Xenos, M.A. and Jankowski, N.J. (in press) Comparing web production practices across electoral web spheres, in R. Kluver, K.A. Foot, N.J. Jankowski and S.M. Schneider (eds), *The Internet and National Elections: A Comparative Study of Web Campaigning*. Cambridge, MA: MIT Press.

Foot, K.A., Schneider, S.M., Xenos, M.A. and Dougherty, M. (in press) Candidates' web practices in the 2002 house, senatorial, and gubernatorial elections. *Journal of Political Marketing*.

Fornäs, J., Klein, K., Ladendorf, M., Sunden, J. and Svenigsson, M. (2002) Into digital borderlands, in J. Fornäs *et al.* (eds) *Digital Borderlands*. New York: Peter Lang, pp. 1–47.

Foster, D. (1997) Community and identity in the electronic village, in D. Holmes (ed.) *Virtual Politics: Identity and Community in Cyberspace*. New York: Sage.

Fox, S. (2004) 'Older Americans and the Internet.' Pew Internet and American Life Project. Available at: www.pewinternet.org/pdfs/PIP_Seniors_Online_2004.pdf.

Franklin, B. (2004) *Packaging Politics: Political Communications in Britain's Media Democracy* (2nd edn). London: Routledge.

Freie, F. (1997) Democratizing the classroom, in G. Reeher and J. Cammarano (eds), *Education for Citizenship*. Lanham, MD: Rowman & Littlefield.

Galbraith, K. (1992) *The Culture of Contentment*. Harmondsworth: Penguin.

Gamson, W. (1988) Political discourse and collective action, in B. Klandermans, H. Kriesi and S. Tarrow (eds) *From Structure to Action: Comparing Social Movement Research Across Cultures*. Greenwich, CT: JAI Press, pp. 219–46.

Garrido, M. and Halavais, A. (2003) Mapping networks of support for the Zapatista movement: applying social-network analysis to study contemporary movements, in M. McCaughey and M. D. Ayers (eds) *Cyberactivism: Online Activism in Theory and Practice*. London: Routledge, pp. 165–84.

Garrido, M. and Halavais, A. (2005) 'Democracy Reloaded: Generation Y and Online Civic Engagement'. Paper presented at the 6th Annual Conference of the Association of Internet Researchers, Chicago, USA, October.

Gerodimos, R. (2006) Democracy and the Internet: access, engagement and deliberation. *Journal of Systemics, Cybernetics, Information, 3*(6), 26–31.

Gibson, R. and McAllister, I. (2006) Does cyber-campaigning win votes? Online communication in the 2004 Australian election. *Journal of Elections, Public Opinions and Parties, 16*(3), 243–63.

Gibson, R. and Ward, S. (2000) A proposed methodology for studying the function and effectiveness of party and candidate web sites. *Social Science Computer Review, 18*(3), 301–19.

Gibson, R., Lusoli, W. and Ward, S. (2002) *UK Political Participation Online: The Public Response. A Survey of Citizens' Political Activity via the Internet.* Salford: ESRI. Available at: www.ipop.org.uk.

Gibson, R. Nixon, P. and Ward, S. (eds) (2003) *Political Parties and the Internet: Net Gain?* London and New York: Routledge.

Giddens, A. (1991) *Modernity and Self Identity.* Cambridge: Polity.

Gidengil, E., Nevitte, A., Blais, N. and Nadeau, N. (2003) Turned off or tuned out? Youth participation in politics. *European Journal of Political Research, 43*(2), 221–36.

Gosling, S. Vazire, S. Srivastva, S. and John, O. (2004) Should we trust web-based studies? A comparative analysis of six preconceptions about internet questionnaires. *American Psychologist, 59*(2), 93–104.

Gould, P. (2003) The empty stadium. *Progressive Politics.* London: Policy Network, vol. 2, no. 3, pp. 68–75.

Graber, D. (2004) Mediated politics and citizenship in the twenty-first century. *Annual Review of Psychology, 55*, 545–71.

Graham, S. (2002) Bridging urban digital divides? *Urban Studies, 39*(1), 33–56.

Gray, M. and Caul, M. (2000) Declining voter turnout in advanced industrial democracies, 1950 to 1997: the effects of declining group mobilization. *Comparative Political Studies, 33*(9), 1091–122.

Grundy, S. and Jamieson, L. (2004) Action, reaction, inaction? Young adults' citizenship in Britain. *Sociologica, 36*(3), 237–52.

Habermas, J. (1989) *The Structural Transformation of the Public Sphere.* Cambridge, MA: MIT Press; Cambridge: Polity Press. (Originally published in German in 1962.)

Hague, B. and Loader, B. (eds) (1999) *Digital Democracy: Discourse and Decision Making in the Information Age.* London and New York: Routledge.

Hajer, M. (2005) *Setting the Stage: A Dramuturgy of Policy Deliberation,* ASSR Working Paper 04/06, Amsterdam School for Social Science Research.

Hammer, T. (1990) *Democracy and the Nation State.* London: Ashgate Publishing.

Hampton, K., and Wellman, B. (2003) Neighboring in netville: how the Internet supports community and social capital in a wired suburb. *City and Community, 2*(4), 277–311.

Hand, M. and Sandywell, B. (2002) E-topia as cosmopolis or citadel. *Theory, Culture & Society, 19*(1–2), 197.

Hansard Society (2001) *None of the Above – Non-Voters and the 2001 Election.* London: Hansard Society.

Hansard Society/Electoral Commission (2004) *Audit of Political Engagement.* London:

Haraway, D. (1985) A cyborg manifesto: science, technology and socialist-feminism in the 1980s. *Socialist Review, 80.*

Hargittai, E. (2004) Internet access and use in context. *New Media and Society, 6*(1), 137–43.

Harris, A. (2001) Revisiting bedroom culture: new spaces for young women's politics. *Hecate, 27*(1), 128–39.

Hassan, R. (2004) *Media, Politics and the Network Society.* Maidenhead: Open University Press.

Haste, H. (2005) *My Voice, My Vote, My Community*. London: Nestle Social Research Programme.

Haythornthwaite, C., and Wellman, B. (2002) The Internet in everyday life: an introduction in B. Wellman and C. Haythornthwaite (eds) *The Internet in Everyday Life*. Oxford: Blackwell, pp. 3–41.

Held, D. (ed.) (2004) *A Globalizing World? Culture, Economics, Politics*. Milton Keynes: Open University Press.

Henn, M., Weinstein, M. and Wring, D. (1999) *Young People and Citizenship: A Study of Opinion in Nottinghamshire*. Nottingham: Nottinghamshire County Council.

Henn, M. Weinstein, M. and Wring, D. (2002) A generation apart? Youth and political participation in Britain. *The British Journal of Politics and International Relations*, 4(2), 167–92.

Hill, A. (2002) *Big Brother*: the real audience. *Television and New Media*, 3(3), 323–40.

Hill, M. and Tisdall, K. (1997) *Children and Society*. London: Longman.

Hillman, K. and Marks, G. (2002) *Becoming an Adult: Leaving Home, Relationships and Home Ownership amongst Australian Youth*. Melbourne: Australian Council for Education Research, Research Report No. 28. Available at: http://www.acer.edu.au/research/LSAY/reports/LSAY28.pdf.

Hoff, J., Horrocks, I. and Tops, P. (eds) (2000) *Democratic Governance and New Technology: Technologically Mediate Innovations in Political Practice in Western Europe*. London and New York: Routledge.

Holden, C. (2004) Heaven help the teachers! Parents' perspectives on the introduction of education for citizenship. *Educational Review*, 56(3), 247–58.

Holmes, D. (ed.) (1997) *Virtual Politics: Identity and Community in Cyberspace*. Sage.

Holsti, O.R. (1969) *Content Analysis for the Social Sciences and Humanities*. Reading, MA: Addison-Wesley.

Horan, P. (1971) Social positions and political cross-pressures: a re-examination. *American Sociological Review*, 36, 650–60.

Howard, P. (2005) Deep democracy, thin citizenship. *Annals of the American Academy of Political and Social Science*, 597, 153–70.

Howland, L. (2002) *Logged Off? How ICT Can Connect Young People and Politics*. London: Demos. Available at: http://www.demos.co.uk/catalogue/loggedoff/.

Inglehart, R. (1977) *The Silent Revolution: Changing Values and Political Styles among Western Publics*. Princeton, NJ: Princeton University Press.

Inspire Foundation (2003) *Reach Out! Website Profiling Research*. Available at: www.inspire.org.au/publications.html.

Inspire Foundation (2004) *2004 Inspire Annual Report*. Available at: www.inspire.org.au/newsannual.html.

Iozzi, D. and Bennett, L. (2005) Crossing the campaign divide: dean changes the election game, in Karen Jagoda (ed.) *Crossing the River: The Coming of Age of the Internet in Politics and Advocacy*. Philadephia, PA: Xlibois.

Istance, D. (2004a) *Knowledge Management in the Learning Society*. Paris: OECD/CERI.

Istance, D. (2004b) *Innovation in the Knowledge Economy: Implications for Education and Learning Systems*. Paris: OECD/CERI.

ITANES (2001) *Perché ha vinto il centro-destra*. Bologna: Il Mulino.

Iyengar, S. and Jackman, S. (2003) 'Technology and Politics: Incentives for Youth Participation.' Paper presented at the International Conference on Civic Education Research, New Orleans, LA, 16–18 November.

Iveson, K. and Scalmer, S. (2000) Contesting the 'inevitable'. *Overland, 161*, 4–13.

Jackson, N. (2004) 'Political parties, their e-newsletters and subscribers: "one night stand" or a "marriage" made in heaven?'. Paper presented at the 54th Annual Conference of the Political Studies Association, London: University of Lincoln, April.

James, A., Jenks, C. and Prout, A. (1998) *Theorizing Childhood*. Cambridge: Cambridge University Press.

Jenkins, Henry and David Thornburn (eds) (2003) *Democracy and New Media*. Cambridge, MA: MIT Press.

Jones, J. (2003) Show your real face: a fan study of the UK *Big Brother* transmissions (2000, 2001, 2002). *New Media and Society, 5*(3): 400–21.

Jones, S. (ed.) (1994) *CyberSociety: Computer-Mediated Communication and Community*. London: Sage.

Jones, S. (ed.) (1997) *Virtual Culture: Identity and Communication in Cybersociety*. London: Sage.

Jones, S. (ed.) (1998) *CyberSociety 2.0: Revisiting Computer-Mediated Communication and Community*. London: Sage.

Jordan, T. (1999) *Cyberpower*. London: Routledge.

Jordan, T. (2002) *Activism!: Direct Action, Hacktivism and the Future of Society*. London: Reaktion.

Jorgensen, C., Kock, C. and Rorbech, L. (1998) Rhetoric that shifts votes: an exploratory study of persuasion in issue-oriented public debates. *Political Communication, 15*(3), 283–99.

Kahn, R. and Kellner, D. (2004) New media and Internet activism: from the 'Battle of Seattle' to blogging. *New Media and Society, 6*(1), 87–95.

Kamarck, E. and Nye, J. (eds) (2002) *Governance.com: Democracy in the Information Age*. Washington, DC: Brookings Institution Press.

Katz, J.E., Rice, R.E. and Aspden, P. (2001) The Internet, 1995–2000. Access, civic involvement, and social interaction. *American Behavioral Scientist, 3*, 405–19.

Keeter, S., Zukin, C., Andolina, M. and Jenkins, K. (2002) *The Civic and Political Health of the Nation: A Generational Portrait*, University of Maryland. Center for Information and Research on Civic Learning and Engagement. Available at: www.puaf.umd.edu/CIRCLE/research/products/Civic_and_Political_Health.pdf.

Kendall, M. (2000) 'Citizenship is Life Long Learning'. Paper presented at IFIP World Computer Congress, Beijing, China, 21–25 August. Available at: www.ifip.org/con2000/iceut2000/iceut01-01.pdf.

Kerr, D., Cleaver, E., White, G. and Judkins, M. (2005) *DCA Connecting with Citizenship Education: A Mapping Study*. Available at: www.nfer.ac.uk//publications/pdfs/downloadable/DMA.PDF.

Kertzer, D. (1988) *Rituals, Politics and Power*. New Haven, CT: Yale University Press.

Kimberlee, R.H. (1998) Young people, the Labour Party and the 1997 General Election. *Renewal, 6*(2), 87–90.

Kimberlee, R.H. (2002) Why don't British young people vote at general elections? *Journal of Youth Studies, 5*(1), 85–98.

Klein, N. (2000) *No Logo: No Space, No Choice, No Jobs*. London: Picador.

Kraut, R., Kiesler, S., Boneva, B., Cummings, J., Helgeson, V. and Crawford, A. (2002). Internet paradox revisited. *Journal of Social Issues, 58*(1), 49–74.

Krueger, B. (2002) Assessing the potential of internet political participation in the United States: a resource approach. *American Politics Research, 30*(5), 476–98.

Lash, S. (2002) *Critique of Information*, London: Sage.

Lawy, R. and Biesta, G. (2006) Citizenship-as-practice. *British Journal of Educational Studies, 54*(1), 34–50.

Leeman, Y. and Ledoux, G. (2003) Preparing teachers for intercultural education. *Teaching Education, 13*(3), 279–92.

Lenhart, A., Fallows, D., and Horrigan, J. (2004) *Content creation online*. Online. Available at: www.pewinternet.org/PPF/r/113/report_display.asp (accessed 20 June 2004).

Lenhart, A., Madden, M. and Hitlin, P. (2005) *Teens and technology: youth are leading the transition to a fully wired and mobile nation*. Online. Available at: www.pewinternet.org/report_display.asp?r=162 (accessed 8 September 2005).

Levine, P. and Lopez, M.H. (2004) *Young People and Political Campaigning on the Internet – Fact Sheet*: The Center for Information and Research on Civic Learning and Engagement, University of Maryland. Available at: www.civic youth.org.

Liff, S., Steward, F. and Watts, P. (2002) New public places for Internet access, in S. Woolgar (ed.), *Virtual Society?* Oxford: Oxford University Press, pp. 78–98.

Lister, R., Smith, N., Middleton, S. and Cox, L. (2003) Young people talk about citizenship: empirical perspectives on theoretical and political debates. *Citizenship Studies, 7*(2), 235–53.

Livingstone, S. (2002) *Young People and New Media: Childhood and the Changing Media Environment*. London: Sage.

Livingstone, S. (2003) Children's use of the internet. *New Media and Society, 5*(2), 147–66.

Livingstone, S. (2004) The challenge of changing audiences: or, what is the audience researcher to do in the age of the Internet. *European Journal of Communication, 19*(1), 75–86.

Livingstone, S. (2005) Critical debates in Internet studies: reflections on an emerging field, in J. Curran and M. Gurevitch (eds) *Mass Media and Society*, 5th edn. London: Sage, pp. 9–28.

Livingstone, S. (2006) Opportunities and constraints framing children and young people's Internet use, in M. Consalvo *et al.* (eds), *Internet Research Annual*, Vol. 4. New York: Peter Lang, pp. 59–75.

Livingstone, S. (in press) The challenge of engaging youth online: contrasting producers' and teenagers' interpretations of websites. *European Journal of Communication, 22*(2).

Livingstone, S. (in press-a) Interactivity and participation on the Internet: A critical appraisal of the online invitation to young people. In P. Dahlgren (ed.), *Young Citizens and New Media: Strategies for Learning Democratic Engagement*.

Livingstone, S. (2007) Youthful experts? A critical appraisal of children's emerging Internet literacy. In C. Ciborra, R. Mansell, D. Quah and R. Silverstone (eds) *Oxford Handbook on ICTs*. Oxford: Oxford University Press.

Livingstone, S. and Bober, M. (2005) *UK Children Go Online: Final Report of Key Project Findings*. London: London School of Economics and Political Science.

Livingstone, S., and Bovill, M. (2001) *Families and the Internet: An Observational Study of Children and Young People's Internet Use. Final Report to BT*. London: London School of Economics.

Livingstone, S. and Helsper, E. (in press). Gradations in digital inclusion: children, young people and the digital divide. *New Media and Society*.

Livingstone, S., Bober, M. and Helsper, E.J. (2005) Active participation or just more information? Young people's take up of opportunities to act and interact on the Internet. *Information, Communication and Society, 8*(3), 287–314.

Lloyd, R. and Bill, A. (2004) *Australia Online: How Australians are Using Computers and the Internet*, ABS Cat. No. 2056. Available at: www.abs.gov.au/Ausstats/abs@.nsf/0/3160d70e0d77b094ca256e18007ddaec?OpenDocument.

Loader, B.D. (ed.) (1997) *The Governance of Cyberspace: Politics, Technology and Global Restructuring*, London: Routledge.

Loader, B.D. (ed.) (1998) *The Cyberspace Divide: Equality, Agency and Policy in the Information Society*, London: Routledge.

Loader, B.D. and Keeble, L. (2004) *Challenging the Digital Divide? A Literature Review of Community Informatics Initiatives*, York: Joseph Rowntree Foundation.

Lock, C., Wright, B., Phillips, T. and Brown. C. (2002) Headroom, promoting the mental health of young people: a multimedia approach. *Youth Studies Australia, 21*(2), 31–5.

Lopez, M.H., Kirby, E. and Sagoff, J. (2005) *The Youth Vote 2004*. Baltimore, MD: University of Maryland, Center for Information and Research on Civic Learning and Engagement.

Lukose, R. (2005) Empty citizenship. *Cultural Anthropology, 20*(4), 506–33.

Lusoli, W., Ward, S. and Gibson, R. (2006) (Re)connecting politics? Parliament, the public and the Internet. *Parliamentary Affairs, 59*(1), 24–42.

McAllister, I. (1997) Political behaviour, in D. Woodward, A. Parkin and J. Summers (eds), *Government, Politics, Power and Policy in Australia*, 6th edn. Melbourne: Longman, pp. 240–68.

McCaughey, M. and Ayers, M.D. (eds) (2003) *Cyberactivism. Online Activism in Theory and Practice*, London: Routledge.

McChesney, R.W. (1996) The Internet and U.S. communication policy-making in historical and critical perspective. *Journal of Communication, 1*, 98–124.

McChesney, R.W. (2000) *Rich Media, Poor Democracy: Communication Politics in Dubious Times*. New York: The New Press.

McCluskey, A. (2004) Schooling: a sustainable learning organisation? ERNIST organisational change study. Berne: CTIE.

McCombs, M. (1997) Building consensus: the news media's agenda-setting roles. *Political Communication, 14*(4), 433–43.

McDonald, M.P. and Popkin, S.L. (2001) The myth of the vanishing voter. *American Political Science Review, 95*(4), 963–74.

McFarlane, A., Williams, J. and Bonnett, M. (2000) Assessment and multimedia authoring. *Journal of Computer Assisted Learning, 16*, 201–12.

MacKenzie, D.A. and Wajcman, J. (eds) (1985) *The Social Shaping of Technology: How the Refrigerator Got Its Hum*. Milton Keynes: Open University Press.

McKuen, M. (1990) Speaking of politics: individual conversational choice, public opinion, and the prospects of deliberative democracy, in J. Ferejohn, and J. Kuklinski (eds) *Information and Democratic Processes*. Urbana, IL: University of Illinois Press, pp. 59–99.

McNeill, L. (1988) *Contradictions of Control*. New York: Routledge.

Madden, M. (2003) *America's Online Pursuits: The Changing Picture of Who's Online and What They Do*. Pew Internet and American Life Project. Available at: www.pewinternet.org/pdfs/PIP_Online_Pursuits_Final.PDF.

Magalhães, A. and Stoer, S. (2003) Performance, citizenship and the knowledge society. *Globalisation, Societies and Education, 1*(1), 41–66.

Magalhães, A. and Stoer, S. (2004) Education, knowledge and the network society. *Globalisation, Societies and Education, 2*(3), 319–35.

Malina, A. (1999) Perspectives on citizen democratisation and alienation in the virtual public sphere, in B. Hague and B. Loader (eds) *Digital Democracy and Decision Making in the Information Age*. London and New York: Routledge.

Manin, B. (1997) *Principles of Representative Government*. Cambridge: Cambridge University Press.

Mannheimer, R. and Sani, G. (2001) *La conquista degli astenuti*. Bologna: Il Mulino.

Mansell, R. (2002) From digital divides to digital entitlements in knowledge societies. *Current Sociology, 50(3)*, 407–26.

Mansell, R. (2004). The Internet, capitalism, and policy, in M. Consalvo, N. Baym, J. Hunsinger, K.B. Jensen, J. Logie, M. Murero and L.R. Shade (eds), *Internet Research Annual*, Vol. 1. New York: Peter Lang, pp. 175–84.

Mantovani, L. and Burnett, S.H. (1998) *The Italian Guillotine: Operation Clean Hands and the Overthrow of Italy's First Republic*. Lanham, MA: Rowman & Littlefield.

Margolis, M. and Resnick, D. (2000) *Politics as Usual: The Cyberspace 'Revolution'*. Thousand Oaks, CA: Sage.

Marshall, T. (1950) *Citizenship and Social Class and Other Essays*. Cambridge: Cambridge University Press.

Martin, M. (2000) *Videoconferencing in teaching and learning: Case studies and guidelines*. Omagh, Northern Ireland: Western Education and Library Board.

Masters, Z., Macintosh, A. and Smith, E. (2004) Young people and e-democracy: creating a culture of participation, in *Proceedings of Third International Conference in E-Government, EGOV 2004*, Zaragoza, Spain, 30 August–3 September.

May, T. (2001) *Social Research: Issues, Methods and Process*, 3rd edn. Buckingham: Open University Press.

Meikle, G. (2002) *Future Active: Media Activism and the Internet*. Sydney: Routledge in cooperation with Pluto Press Australia.

Meyer, D. and Staggenborg, S. (1996) Movements, countermovements, and the structure of political opportunity. *The American Journal of Sociology, 101*(6), 1628–60.

Millard, E. (1997) *Differently Literate: Boys, Girls and the Schooling of Literacy*. London: Falmer.

Miller, A., Wattenberg M. and Malunchuk, O. (1986) Schematic assessments of presidential candidates. *American Political Science Review, 80*, 521–40.

Milliken, M. (2001) Building bridges through the web. *The Development Education Journal, 7*(2), 8–11.

Monge, P.R. (2004) 'History and Emergence of Communication Networks.' Networkshop. International Communication Association. New Orleans, 27 May.

Montgomery, K. (2001) The new on-line children's consumer culture, in D. Singer and J. Singer (eds) *Handbook of Children and the Media*. London: Sage, pp. 635–50.

Montgomery, K., Gottlieg-Robles, B. and Larson, G.O. (2004) *Youth as E-Citizens: Engaging the Digital Generation*, Center for Social Media, School of Communication, American University. Available at: www.centerforsocialmedia.org/ecitizens/youthreport.pdf (accessed 9 April 2004).

MORI (2004) *The Rules of Engagement? Participation, Involvement and Voting in Britain: Research Analysis for the Electoral Commission and the Hansard Society.* London: MORI.

Morris, P. and Cogan, J. (2001) A comparative overview: Civic education across six societies. *International Journal of Educational Research, 35*, 109–23.

Morris, Z., John P. and Halpern, D. (2003) Compulsory citizenship for the disenfranchised. *The Curriculum Journal, 14*(2): 1–19.

Mossberger, K., Tolbert, C. and Stansbury, M. (2003) *Virtual Inequality*. Washington, DC: Georgetown University Press.

Mouffe, C. (ed.) (1992) *Dimensions of Radical Democracy: Pluralism, Citizenship, Community*, London: Verso.

Mulgan, G. and Wilkinson, H. (1997) Freedom's children and the rise of generational politics, in G. Mulgan (ed.) *Life after Politics: New Thinking for the Twenty-first Century.* London: Fontana Press.

Murdock, G. and Golding, P. (1989) Information poverty and political inequality: citizenship in the age of privatized communication. *Journal of Communication, 39*(3), 180–95.

Mutz, D. (2002) The consequences of cross-cutting networks for political participation. *American Journal of Political Science, 46*(4), 838–55.

Mutz, D. (2004) Leading horses to water: Confessions of a *Daily Show* junkie. *Journalism and Mass Communication Educator, 59*, 31–5.

Newman, J., Barnes, M., Sullivan, H. and Knops, A. (2004) Public participation and collaborative governance. *Journal of Social Policy, 33*, 203–23.

New Voter Project (2004) *Youth Vote Drove Turnout Increase in 2004 Election*. Available at: www.newvotersproject.org/youth_turnout_increase.

Niens, U. and O'Connor, U. (2005) Evaluation of the Introduction of Local and Global Citizenship to the Northern Ireland Curriculum. Interim report to CCEA, September.

Nixon, P. and Johansson, H. (1999) Transparency through technology: the Internet and political participation, in B. Hague and B. Loader (eds) *Digital Democracy: Discourse and Decision Making in the Information Age*. London and New York: Routledge.

Norris, P. (2001) *Digital Divide. Civic Engagement, Information Poverty and the Internet Worldwide*. Cambridge: Cambridge University Press.

Norris, P. (2002) *Democratic Phoenix: Reinventing Political Activism*. Cambridge: Cambridge University Press.

Norris, P. (2003) Preaching to the converted? Pluralism, participation and party websites. *Party Politics, 9(1)*, 21–45.

Northern Ireland Office (2006) Available at: www.nio.gov.uk/index/key-issues.htm (accessed 4 May 2006).

O'Connor, U., Hartop, B. and McCully, A. (2002) 'A review of the Schools Community Relations Programme 2002', a consultation document published by the Department of Education for Northern Ireland.

Ofcom (2005) *Viewers and Voters: Attitudes to Television Coverage of the 2005 General Election*. London: Office of Communications.

Ofcom (2006) *Media Literacy Audit: Report on Adult Media Literacy.* London: Office of Communications.

OFM (2005) *A Shared Future. Policy and Strategic Framework for Good Relations in Northern Ireland.* Belfast: Office of the First Minister and Deputy First Minister, March.

OfSTED (2003) *Implementation of National Curriculum Citizenship.* London: Office for Standards in Education.

OfSTED (2005) *An Evaluation of the Post-16 Citizenship Pilot 2004/05.* London: Office for Standards in Education.

Olssen, M. (2004) From the Crick Report to the Parekh Report. *British Journal of Sociology of Education, 25*(2), 179–92.

Olsson, T. (2002) *Mycket väsen om ingenting: hur datorn och Internet undgår att formas till medborgarens tekniker.* [Much ado about nothing: how the computer and the Internet miss their plight as tools for the citizen] PhD thesis. AUU, Uppsala Studies in Media and Communication.

Olsson, T. (2004) *Oundgängliga resurser: Om medier, IKT och lärande bland partipolitiskt aktiva ungdomar.* [Indispensable resources: on media, ICTs and learning among young, politically active people]. Lund: Department of Sociology, Lund University.

Olsson, T. (2005a) Young citizens, ICTs and learning. A design for a study of the media and political activity. *Nordicom Review, 26*(1), 131–40.

Olsson, T. (2005b) *Alternativa resurser: Om medier, IKT och lärande bland ungdomar i alternativa rörelser.* [Alternative resources: On media, ICTs and learning among young, alternative people]. Lund: Department of Sociology, Lund University.

Olsson, T. (2006) Appropriating civic information and communication technology: a critical study of Swedish ICT-policy visions. *New Media and Society, 8*(4), 611–27.

Ornstein, N.J. and Mann, T.E. (2000) *The Permanent Campaign and its Future*, Washington, DC: American Enterprise Institute and The Brookings Institution.

O'Toole, T., Lister, M., Marsh, D., Jones, S. and McDonagh, A. (2003) Tuning out or left out? Participation and non-participation among young people. *Contemporary Politics, 9*(1), 45–61.

Oulton, C., Day, V., Dillon, J. and Grace, M. (2004) Controversial issues: teachers' attitudes and practices in the context of citizenship education. *Oxford Review of Education, 30*(4), 489–507.

Pammett, J. and LeDuc (2003) *Explaining the Turnout in Canadian Federal Elections: A New Survey of Non-Voters.* Ottawa: Elections Canada.

Park, H.W. (2003) Hyperlink network analysis: a new method for the study of social structure on the web. *Connections, 25*(1), 49–61.

Pattie, C.J., Seyd, P. and Whiteley, P. (2004) *Citizenship in Britain: Values, Participation and Democracy.* Cambridge: Cambridge University Press.

Pew (2001) *Teenage Life Online: the Rise of the Instant-Message Generation and the Internet's Impact on Friendships and Family Relationships*: Pew Internet and American Life Project. Available at: www.pewInternet.org.

Pew (2002) *One Year Later: September 11 and the Internet.* Washington, DC: Pew Internet and American Life Project. Available at: www.pewInternet.org.

Pew (2004a) *Pew Research Center Biennial News Consumption Survey.* Available at: www.people-press.org/reports/pdf/.

Pew (2004b) *Young People More Engaged, More Uncertain, Debates More Important to Young Voters*. Pew Internet and American Life Project. Available at: www. pewinternet.org. Available at://peoplepress.org/commentary/display.php3?Analysis ID=99.

Pew (2005) *A Decade of Adoption: How the Internet has woven itself into American life*. Washington, DC: Pew Internet and American Life. Available at: www. pewinternet.org.

Phipps, L. (2000) New communications technologies: a conduit for social inclusion. *Information, Communication and Society, 3*(1), 39–68.

Pickerill, J. (2003) *Cyberprotest. Environmental Activism Online*, Manchester: Manchester University Press.

Pollak, A. (2006) Educational co-operation on the island of Ireland: are the good years ending? *The Journal of Cross Border Studies, 1*, Spring, 34–48.

Porter, D. (ed.) (1997) *Internet Culture*. London: Routledge.

Poster, M. (1997) Cyberdemocracy: Internet and the public sphere, in D. Porter (ed.) *Internet Culture*. London and New York: Routledge.

Postman, N. (1987) *Amusing Ourselves to Death*, London: Methuen.

Power (2006) *The Report of Power: An Independent Inquiry into Britain's Democracy*. London: Joseph Rowntree Foundation.

Productivity Commission (2003) *Social Capital: Reviewing the Concept and its Policy Implications*. Canberra: Ausinfo, Research paper. Available at: www.pc.gov.au/ research/commres/socialcapital/index.html.

Prout, A. (2000) Children's participation: control and self-realisation in British late modernity. *Children and Society, 14(3)*, 304–15.

Putnam, R.D. (2000) *Bowling Alone: The Collapse and Revival of American Community*. New York: Simon & Schuster.

QCA (1998) *Education for Citizenship and the Teaching of Democracy in Schools*. London: QCA.

Quan-Haase, A. and Wellman, B. (2002) *How Does the Internet Affect Social Capital*. Available at: www.chass.utoronto.ca/~wellman/publications/index.html.

Quan-Haase, A., Wellman, B., Witte, J. and Hampton, K. (2002) Capitalizing on the net: social contact, civic engagement, and the sense of community, in B. Wellman and C. Haythornthwaite (eds) *The Internet in Everyday Life*. Oxford: Blackwell Publishing.

Qvortrup, J. (1995) Childhood and modern society: a paradoxical relationship, in J. Brannen and M. O'Brien (eds) *Childhood and Parenthood*. London: Institute of Education, University of London, pp. 189–98.

Rahn, W.M. and Transue, J.E. (1998) Social trust and value change: the decline of social capital in American youth, 1976–1995. *Political Psychology, 19*(3), 545–64.

Rainie, L. and Horrigan, J. (2005) *A Decade of Adoption: How the Internet Has Woven Itself Into American Life*. Available at: www.pewinternet.org/PPF/r/148/ report_display.asp> (accessed 14 February, 2005).

Rainie, L., Cornfield, M. and Horrigan, J. (2005) *The Internet and Campaign 2004*. Pew Internet and American Life Project Report. Available at: www.pewInternet. org/pdfs/PIP_2004_Campaign.pdf.

Roberts, J. (2004) Some Everyday Experiences of Voluntarism. *Social Politics, 11*(2): 280–96.

Rassool, N. (1999) Flexible identities. *British Journal of Sociology of Education, 20*(1), 23–36.

Risinger, F. (1997) Citizenship education and the world wide web. *Social Education, 61*(4), 223–4.

Robinson, J.P. and Levy, M.R. (1986) *The Main Source: Learning from Television News*. Beverly Hills, CA: Sage.

Roker, D., Player, K. and Coleman, J. (1999) Young people's voluntary and campaigning activities as sources of political education. *Oxford Review of Education, 25*(1/2), 185–98.

Rossiter, N. (2004) 'Organized networks'. Paper presented at The Life of Mobile Data: Technology, Mobility and Data Subjectivity, University of Surrey, April.

Sanders, D. (2002) Behaviouralism, in D. Marsh and G. Stoker (eds) *Theory and Methods in Political Science*, 2nd edn. Basingstoke: Palgrave, pp. 45–64.

Sanders, L. (2001) 'The Psychological Benefits of Political Participation'. Paper presented at the Annual Meeting of the American Political Science Association, San Francisco.

Scalmer, S. (2002) *Dissent Events*. Sydney: UNSW Press.

Scammell, M. (2000) The internet and civic engagement. *Political Communication, 17*(4), 351–5.

Schier, S. (2000) *By Invitation Only: The Rise of Exclusive Politics in the United States*, Pittsburgh, PA: Pittsburgh University Press.

Schweisfurth, M. (2006) Education for global citizenship. *Educational Review, 58*(1), 41–50.

Scullion, R. and Dermody, J. (2005) The strategic value of party election broadcasts: a content analysis of the 2001 British general election campaign. *International Journal of Advertising, 24*(3), 345–72.

Selwyn, N. (2003) The impact of mobile technologies on schools and schooling. *British Journal of Sociology of Education, 24*(2), 131–43.

Selwyn, N. (2004) Reconsidering political and popular understandings of the digital divide. *New Media and Society, 6*(3), 341–62.

Sennett, R. (1978) *The Fall of Public Man*. New York: Alfred A. Knopf.

Sennett, R. (2006) *The Culture of the New Capitalism*. New Haven, CT and London: Yale University Press.

Shah, D., Kwak, N. and Holbert, L. (2001) 'Connecting' and 'disconnecting' with civic life: patterns of Internet use and the production of social capital. *Political Communication, 18*(2), 141–62.

Shane, P. (ed.) (2004) *Democracy Online: The Prospects for Political Renewal Through the Internet*. London: Routledge.

Shelley, M., Thrane, L., Shulman, S., Lang, E. and Beisser, S. *et al.* (2004) Digital citizenship. *Social Science Computer Review, 22*(2), 1–14.

Simon, A. and Xenos, M. (2000) Media framing and effective public deliberation. *Political Communication, 17*(4), 363–76.

Singer, J. B. and Gonzalez-Verez, M. (2003) Envisioning the caucus community: online newspaper editors conceptualize their political roles. *Political Communication, 20*, 433–52.

Slater, D. (2002) Social relationships and identity online and offline, in L. Lievrouw and S. Livingstone (eds) *The Handbook of New Media*. London: Sage.

Smith, A. and Robinson, A. (1996) *Education for Mutual Understanding: The Initial Statutory Years*. Centre for the Study of Conflict, University of Ulster, pp. 77–8.

Smith, C.A. and Smith, K.B. (2000) A rhetorical perspective on the 1997 British party manifestos. *Political Communication, 17*(4), 457–73.

Smith, J., Kearns, M. and Fine, A. (2005) *Power to the Edges: Trends and Opportunities in Online Civic Engagement.* Online. Available at: www.evolvefoundation. org/files/Pushing_Power_to_the_Edges_05–06–05.pdf (accessed 30 August 2005).

Soysal, Y. (1998) Citizenship and identity: living in indiasporas in post-war Europe? *Ethnic and Racial Studies, 23*(1), 1–15.

Stanyer, J. (2005) The British public and political attitude expression: the emergence of a self-expressive political culture? *Contemporary Politics, 11*(1), 19–32.

Stevenson, N. (2000) The future of public media cultures. *Information, Communication and Society, 3*(2), 192–214.

Street, J. (1997) *Politics and Popular Culture.* Cambridge: Polity Press.

Stromer-Galley, J. (2000) On-line interaction and why candidates avoid it. *Journal of Communication, 50*(4), 111–32.

Stromer-Galley, J. and Foot, K.A. (2002) Citizen perceptions of online interactivity and implications for political campaign communication. *Journal of Computer-Mediated Communication, 8(1).* Available at: http://jcmc.indiana.edu/vol8/issue1/ stromerandfoot.html (accessed 14 May 2007).

Subrahmanyam, K., Greenfield, P., Kraut, R. and Gross, E. (2001) The impact of computer use on children's and adolescents' development. *Journal of Applied Developmental Psychology, 22*(1), 7–30.

Sundar, S.S., Kalyanaraman, S. and Brown, J. (2003) Explicating Web site interactivity: Impresssion formation effects in political campaign sites. *Communication Research, 30*(1), 30–59.

Sundberg, P.A. (2001) Building Positive Attitudes Among Geographically Diverse Students: The Project 1–57 Experience. Boston, MA: National Educational Computing Conference, 'Building on the Future', 25–27 July.

Sunstein, C. (2003) *Why Societies Need Dissent.* Boston, MA: Harvard University Press.

Supple, C. (1999) Ideals for citizenship education. *Multicultural Teaching, 18*(1), 16–19.

Tewksbury, D. (2003) What do Americans really want to know? Tracking the behaviour of news readers on the Internet. *Journal of Communication, 53*(4), 694–710.

The 2004 Presidential Election and Young Voters (2004) *Center for Information and Research on Civic Learning and Engagement Fact Sheet.* Updated October 28, 2004. Available at: www.civicyouth.org/PopUps/FactSheets/FS_04_Poll_ Summary.pdf.

The Youth Vote 2004 (2004) Center for Information and Research on Civic Learning and Engagement Fact Sheet. Available at: www.civicyouth.org/PopUps/FactSheets/ FS_Youth_Voting_72–04.pdf.

Tolbert, C. and McNeal, R. (2003) Unraveling the effects of the Internet on political participation. *Political Research Quarterly,* 56: 175–85.

Tops, P., Voerman, G. and Boogers, M. (2000) Political websites during the 1998 parliamentary elections in the Netherlands, in J. Hoff, I. Horrocks and P. Tops (eds) *Democratic Governance and New Technology: Technologically Mediated Innovations in Political Practice in Western Europé.* London and New York: Routledge/ECPR Studies in European Political Science.

Touraine, A. (2000) *Can We Live Together?* Cambridge: Polity.

Turkle, S. (1995) *Life on the Screen: Identity in the Age of the Internet.* New York: Simon & Schuster.

Urry, J. (2000) *Sociology beyond Societies: Mobilities for the Twenty First Century*, London: Routledge.

Urry, J. (2003) *Global Complexity*. Cambridge: Polity.

van de Donk, W., Loader, B.D., Nixon, P.G. and Rucht, D. (eds) (2004) *Cyberprotest. New Media, Citizens and Social Movements*, New York and London: Routledge.

van Zoonen, L. (2004) Imagining the fan democracy. *European Journal of Communication, 19*(1), 39–52.

Verba, S., Schlozman, K.L. and Brady, H.E. (1995) *Voice and Equality: Civic Voluntarism in American Politics*. Cambridge, MA: Cambridge University Press.

Vibewire (2004) *Vibewire Youth Services Annual Report 2003-2004*. Provided via personal communication with Vibewire.

Vibewire (2005) Young people and media: Opposite sides of the fence? Prepared by Simon Moss, Dee Jefferson and Dinah Arndt. Provided via personal communication with Vibewire,

Volti, R. (1992) *Society and Technological Change*. New York: St Martin's Press.

Vromen, A. (2003) People try to put us down: participatory citizenship of 'Generation X'. *Australian Journal of Political Science, 38*(1), 78–99.

Vromen, A. and Gelber, K. (2005) *Powerscape: Contemporary Australian Political Practice*. Sydney: Allen & Unwin.

Wagner, G. (2000) There never was internet sociology, in R. Rogers (ed.), *Preferred Placement*. Maastricht: Jan van Eyck Akademie.

Ward, S. and Lusoli, W. (2003) Dinosaurs in cyberspace? British trade unions and the Internet. *European Journal of Communication, 18(2)*, 147–79.

Ward, S. and Lusoli, W. (2003) Logging on or switching off? in S. Coleman and S. Ward (eds) *Spinning the Web*, London: Hansard Society, pp. 13–22.

Ward, S., Gibson, R. and Lusoli, W. (2003) Participation and mobilisation online: hype, hope and reality. *Parliamentary Affairs, 56*(3), 652–68.

Ward, S., Gibson, R. and Lusoli, W. (2005) 'Old Politics, New Media: Parliament, the Public and the Internet'. Paper presented at the 55th Annual Conference of the Political Studies Association, University of Leeds, April.

Warkentin, C. (2001) *Reshaping World Politics. NGOs, the Internet and Global Civil Society*. Lanham, MA: Rowman & Littlefield.

Weare, C. and Lin, W.Y. (2000) Content analysis of the World Wide Web: opportunities and challenges. *Social Science Computer Review, 18*(3), 272–92.

Weaver, D.H, Zhu, J.-H. and Willnat, L. (1992) The bridging function of interpersonal communication in agenda–setting. *Journalism Quarterly, 69*(4), 856–67.

Webster, F. (2001) *Theories of the Information Society*, London: Routledge.

Wellman, B. and Hampton, K. (1999) Living networked on and offline. *Contemporary Sociology, 28*(6), 648–54.

Wellman, B. and Haythornthwaite, C. (2002) *The Internet in Everyday life*. Malden, MA: Blackwell.

Wellman, B., Quan Haase, A., Witte, J. and Hampton, K. (2001) Does the Internet increase, decrease, or supplement social capital? Social networks, participation, and community commitment. *American Behavioral Scientist, 3*: 436–55.

Wenger, E. (1998) *Communities of Practice*. Cambridge: Cambridge University Press.

Westheimer, J. and Kahne, J. (2004) What kind of citizen? *American Educational Research Journal, 41*(2), 237–69.

White, N. (2006) *Facilitating and Hosting a Virtual Community*. Available online at: www.fullcirc.com (accessed 16 January 2006).

White, R. and Wyn, J. (2004) *Youth and Society: Exploring the Social Dynamics of Youth Experience*. Melbourne: Oxford University Press.

Wilhelm, A. (2000) *Democracy in the Digital Age: Challenges to Political Life in Cyberspace*. London and New York: Routledge.

Williams, A.P., Trammell, K.D., Postelnicu, M., Landreville, K.D., and Martin, J.D. (2005) Blogging and hyperlinking: Use of the Web to enhance viability during 2004 U.S. campaigns. *Journalism Studies*, 6(2), 177–86.

Williams, R. and Edge, D. (1996) The social shaping of technology, in W.H. Dutton (ed.), *Information and Communication Technologies: Visions and Realities*. Oxford: Oxford University Press, pp. 53–68.

Willson, M. (1997) Community in the abstract: a political and ethical dilemma?' in D. Holmes (ed.) *Virtual Politics: Identity and Community in Cyberspace*. London: Sage.

Winston, B. (1996) *Media Technology and Society: A History – From the Telegraph to the Internet*. London: Routledge.

Winter, I. (2000) Major themes and debates in the social capital literature: the Australian context, in Ian Winter (ed.) *Social Capital and Public Policy in Australia*. Melbourne: Australian Institute of Family Studies, pp. 17–42.

Woolgar, S. (2002) Five rules of virtuality, in S. Woolgar (ed.) *Virtual Society? Technology, Cyberbole, Reality*. Oxford: Oxford University Press, pp. 1–22).

Wyn, J. and White, R. (1997) *Rethinking Youth*. Sydney: Allen & Unwin.

Youth Voting in the 2004 Election (2004) *Center for Information and Research on Civic Learning and Engagement Fact Sheet*. Updated November 8, 2004. Available at: www.civicyouth.org/PopUps/FactSheets/FS-PresElection04.pdf.

Zhao, W., Massey, B. L., Murphy, J. and Fang, L. (2003) Cultural dimensions of website design and content. *Prometheus, 21*(1), 75–84.

Index

Page references in italics indicate illustrations.

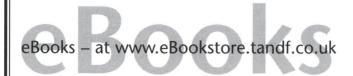